Team-Based Shared Formulation for Psychosis

Adding to the growing literature on shared formulation, the authors provide over two decades of practice-based evidence for the use of a Shared Assessment, Formulation and Education (SAFE) approach to working with those with complex mental health and behavioural needs.

The SAFE approach offers an evidence-informed framework for multidisciplinary teams to address the needs of those with complex and enduring psychosis for whom current evidence-based interventions are ineffective in promoting their recovery. Drawing from richly detailed case studies, the authors provide a range of useful tools and formulation templates for use by clinicians and professionals alike. They put forward a shared language to promote a multidisciplinary understanding of service users' complex needs and a means of organising treatment into a focused, realistic and targeted approach aimed at reducing barriers to recovery and allowing individuals to lead personally meaningful lives. The book focuses predominantly on the treatment of those with psychosis who require bespoke, multi-theory informed care.

This work will be an invaluable resource to professionals working with this client group, including clinical and counselling psychologists, psychiatrists and other allied health professionals.

Alan Meaden is a consultant clinical psychologist with over 25 years of experience working in designing and researching rehabilitation services. He formed part of the leading research team in the development of cognitive-behavioural approaches to command hallucinations and has published extensively in this area. Throughout this period, he continued to work as a clinician developing clinical insights through his work with service users, their families and the teams that supported them. After retiring from managing a substantial NHS psychology service, he continues to work as a freelance consultant, supervisor and trainer.

Andrew Fox is a clinical psychologist working across inpatient recovery and rehabilitation services. He is also a lecturer in the Centre for Applied Psychology at the University of Birmingham. Much of his work involves trying to develop an understanding of the psychology of complex mental health needs in an effort to enhance well-being.

Henna Hussain is a clinical psychologist currently working for Birmingham and Solihull Mental Health NHS Foundation Trust. Henna works in both a Community Mental Health Team and in Recovery and Rehabilitation inpatient services. Prior to this, she worked for two years in addiction services within the same trust.

'Improving the recovery and quality of life for people with psychosis is nearly always a team-based responsibility: whether in early intervention, assertive outreach, rehabilitation or generic mental health teams. I have always been struck by the differences between teams with the same function in their capacity to absorb and manage risk safely without jeopardising their fundamental mission to care, empower and promote recovery and well-being. I've never quite been able to put my finger on why teams differ in this way; perhaps leadership, structure, model fidelity, expectations, etc., let alone how to work with a whole team to hit the sweet spot. Alan Meaden, Andrew Fox and Henna Hussain have dedicated over two decades' work to this task with spectacular results. In this book they demonstrate with clarity and accessible case material their approach built on a *team-based shared formulation*, and how it can provide a solid foundation for interventions delivered by the whole team, such as relapse prevention, easing distress from the troubled internal world, through to social recovery. This is the key to the successful translation of evidence-based interventions through a team platform and is *essential* reading for all psychosis teams. I cannot recommend it highly enough.'

Max Birchwood, Professor of Youth Mental Health
at Warwick Medical School, University of Warwick

Team-Based Shared Formulation for Psychosis

The SAFE Approach

Alan Meaden, Andrew Fox
and Henna Hussain

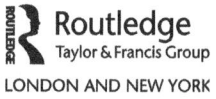
Routledge
Taylor & Francis Group

LONDON AND NEW YORK

Cover image: © Image Source/Getty Images

First published 2023
by Routledge
4 Park Square, Milton Park, Abingdon, Oxon OX14 4RN

and by Routledge
605 Third Avenue, New York, NY 10158

Routledge is an imprint of the Taylor & Francis Group, an informa business

British Library Cataloguing-in-Publication Data
A catalogue record for this book is available from the British Library

Library of Congress Cataloging-in-Publication Data
A catalog record for this book has been requested

ISBN: 978-0-367-53668-8 (hbk)
ISBN: 978-0-367-53667-1 (pbk)
ISBN: 978-1-003-08281-1 (ebk)

DOI: 10.4324/9781003082811

Typeset in Times New Roman
by Apex CoVantage, LLC

Contents

List of Appendices   vii
List of Figures   viii
List of Tables   ix
Acknowledgements   x
Note on the Cover Image   xi
List of Abbreviations   xii

Introduction   1

1 Understanding Risk and Problematic Behaviour in Psychosis   4

2 Getting Started: Assessing and Formulating the Team and
  the Service   16

3 Shared Formulation: Principles and Practice in SAFE   28

4 Risk Assessment in SAFE   38

5 Using Early Warning Signs in SAFE   57

6 CARM Revisited   72

7 Planning and Delivering Behavioural Interventions in SAFE   92

8 Using TBCT to Modify the Person's Internal World   105

9 Intervening Across Internal and External Domains of the
  Person's World   126

10 Using Multiple Shared Formulations to Inform Care
    Planning and Intervention   142

11 Applying SAFE to Other Settings   160

12 Measuring Outcomes and Capturing Change   175

    Concluding Remarks   189

    Appendices   192
    References   204
    Index   219

Appendices

1   Service Level Formulation Template   194
2   CARM Template for Active Behaviours   196
3   CARM Template for Passive Behaviours   197
4   Static-Dynamic Risk Formulation and Care Plan   198
5   Challenging Behaviour Record Sheet for Psychosis (CBRS-P)   199
6   Resettlement Scale   200

Figures

3.1   The Cognitive ABC Formulation   32

6.1   Timothy's CARM for Inappropriate Questions and Sexual Remarks   80

6.2   Sandra's CARM for Passive Behaviours   86

6.3   CARM-Informed Service User and Staff ABC   90

8.1   CARM Formulation of Luke Not Using a Mobile Phone   124

11.1   Emma's CARM for Taking an Overdose   170

Tables

1.1	ABC Formulation	14
4.1	Evidence-Based START Strength and Vulnerability Items for Each Area	46
5.1	Rakeem's Team-Based Stress Management Plan	61
5.2	Steve's EWS-R Plan for Physical Violence Towards Others (e.g. punching, hitting)	69
7.1	Paul's PBS Plan	98
7.2	Paul's CBRS-P^{PBS}	100
8.1	Steve's ABC	112
8.2	Steve's Staff's ABC	113
8.3	Steve's ABC TBCT Plan	114
10.1	Steve's SLF	145
10.2	Steve's SMART Goal for Community Integration	146
10.3	Steve's START Items for Key and Critical Areas	147
10.4	Steve's Static-Dynamic Risk Formulation and Care Plan – Physical Assault (with or without weapons)	152
10.5	Otis's Key and Critical Area Items for Substance Use and Suicide	156
10.6	Otis's Static-Dynamic Risk Formulation and Care Plan	157
10.7	Otis's SMART Goal for Developing a Social Network	158
11.1	Richard's Team-Based Safety Plan	166
11.2	Emma's EWS-R Plan for Taking Overdoses	171
12.1	Linking Assessment Recommendations to Care Plan Monitoring	179
12.2	Jocelyn's Service Level Reformulation Changes	183
12.3	Changes in START Areas	185
12.4	Changes in START Item-Rating Supporting Evidence	186

Acknowledgements

I would like to thank my colleague, mentor and friend Max Birchwood for all his support and words of wisdom over the past 25 years. Max, you are a true pioneer. Also, I would like to thank my co-authors Andy and Henna for joining me on this part of the SAFE journey and for their ideas and insights and for always having my back. Last but by no means least, I would like to thank my wife Ann for her unswerving support and love over many, many years.

Alan Meaden, November 2021

I would like to thank Alan for his wise counsel and sage advice over all the years and Henna for her enthusiasm, fresh ideas and keen ability to keep Alan and me on track during book meetings. Also, I would like to thank my family, friends and colleagues for the understanding and kindness I have been fortunate to be shown.

Andrew Fox, November 2021

I would like to express my heartfelt gratitude to both Alan and Andy for allowing me to join them in their amazing journey. I have learnt so much from you both and I am still in awe of not only the knowledge and wisdom that you both possess but in the overall kindness, generosity, creativity and passion that I have had the pleasure of witnessing throughout our time together. You both really do care about the people we work for, and it's been amazing to see how you advocate fiercely for this population group. I would also like to say a big thank you to my family and friends for their support, patience and understanding for those times when I couldn't always be there.

Henna Hussain, November 2021

The authors also collectively acknowledge the kind permission given by Taylor and Francis for the republication of material contained within Appendix 5: Copyright (© 2011) From *Problematic and Risk Behaviours in Psychosis: A Shared Formulation Approach* by Alan Meaden and David Hacker. Reproduced by permission of Taylor and Francis Group, LLC, a division of Informa plc.

Note on the Cover Image

The hedgerow symbolises the team. A good team takes time to evolve. It is an organic ecosystem. Like the hedgerow, it has many different elements that learn to coexist and support each other. It grows together slowly and cannot be quickly assembled simply by occupying the same space. When established, it is strong and can resist external forces. Some elements of the hedgerow stick out to seek their own space but remain firmly attached. They provide the basis for the hedgerow to expand and continue growing. Teams define the landscape of care. Like the hedgerow, teams need regular maintenance and care if they are not to wither and die.

With much gratitude to Peter Hulme (retired Consultant Lead Psychologist for Rehabilitation Services – Hereford) for sharing the initial idea.

Abbreviations

AOT	Assertive Outreach Team
CARM	Cognitive Approach to Risk Management
CBC-P	Challenging Behaviour Checklist for Psychosis
CBRS-P	Challenging Behaviour Record Sheet for Psychosis
CBT-P	Cognitive Behaviour Therapy for Psychosis
CRU	Community Rehabilitation Unit
EWS-P	Early Warning Signs of Psychotic relapse
EWS-R	Early Warning Signs of Risk
GAST	Goal Attainment Scaling Tool
HDU	High Dependency Unit
MDT	Multidisciplinary Team
PBS	Positive Behaviour Support Plan
RRES	Residential Rehabilitation Engagement Scale
RS	Resettlement Scale
SAFE	Shared Assessment, Formulation and Education
SLF	Service Level Shared Formulation
SPJ	Structured Professional Judgment
TBCT	Team Based Cognitive Therapy
WHO	World Health Organization

Introduction

Meaden and Hacker (2010) made the case for an integrated multidisciplinary approach underpinned by cognitive-behavioural theory and practice, embedded within a shared formulation framework and guided by need-adapted (Alanen, 1997) principles. This approach we called the Shared Assessment Formulation and Education (SAFE). It was developed to better meet the needs of people who experience psychosis as part of complex mental health and behavioural needs and can be hard to reach. The three boroughs trilogy of studies mapped these needs for a cohort of over 100 service users over the course of a decade (Cowan et al., 2012; Edwards et al., 2022; Meaden et al., 2014). They reveal a pattern of high service utilisation and poor functional outcomes associated with problem behaviours and poor engagement. Clearly, despite changes brought about in healthcare delivery in the UK, there remains a group for whom existing mainstream services and interventions are often ineffective and who consequently require high levels of support, often in detained settings. Ten years on, it seems that further innovation is needed to meet the complex needs of this particular group. Increasing the availability and quality of established interventions alone is unlikely to help, particularly given that interventions such as Cognitive Behaviour Therapy for Psychosis (CBT-P) yield somewhat disappointing results (Reid, 2019). Risk and challenging behaviours often severely limit the individual's independence and freedom, significantly reducing their ability to access such treatments.

One set of issues to emerge is the failure of outcome studies, and correspondingly, services, to target and measure the most relevant factors (Birchwood & Trower, 2006). In the first of the series of studies carried out across three boroughs of the West Midlands, Cowan et al. (2012) conducted a survey of the clinical characteristics of service users in ten 24-hour NHS nursing care facilities. Of the total 108 inpatients, data were obtained for 98. This population was characterised by significant use of inpatient services over a long period, having active psychotic symptoms, poor social functioning and being deemed unsuitable for independent living, despite interventions over a prolonged period. Substantial numbers had recent aggression, especially those in locked units who also had a history of serious violence.

DOI: 10.4324/9781003082811-1

In the second study, Meaden et al. (2014) explicitly assessed engagement and problem behaviours in this same population. The poor levels of engagement reported were striking, especially in regard to actively participating in treatments. The lack of therapeutic engagement is of particular concern, particularly when considering the widespread problematic behaviours reported not only concerning behaviours required for independent living ("failure to perform a range of everyday activities") but also the persistently high levels of verbal aggression and socially inappropriate behaviours. These make placement outside of a nursing care setting difficult and together with systemic issues, such as the restricted availability of suitable community alternatives, may explain a lack of discharge for this group. The lack of engagement in discussion of symptoms and behaviours suggests that individuals did not share the view that these were important factors to be understood and managed. A lack of shared understanding increases the possibility that while such problematic issues may be managed through relational security and interpersonal monitoring, there is a risk of these re-emerging if discharged to a less supervised setting. Whilst there remains a role for standard CBT-P as well as other psychological interventions and psychologically informed environments with those who are better able to discuss their experiences and become actively involved in their treatment, for this population this is unlikely to be successful. One hopeful finding of the Meaden et al. (2014) study was the much higher levels of engagement shown across all service types with the named nurse; possibly because of their ability to meet the service users' fundamental needs (e.g. accessing leave, help with practical activities). This affords an opportunity to utilise interventions that can be delivered by the team in the context of these relationships. Such existing therapeutic relationships can be nurtured to facilitate a focus on problematic behaviours as barriers to personal recovery. Importantly, we advocate a shift away from emphasising engagement at the exclusion of recognising that this occurs in the context of a two-way (at least) relationship, with responsibilities for all parties. This shifts the focus of rehabilitative interventions away from symptoms or disabilities and redirects the goal towards building relationships and managing problematic behaviours. A further implication of these findings is the need to routinely assess engagement and problematic behaviours utilising them both as individual measures and for service evaluation purposes.

In the final study ten years later, Edwards et al. (2022) were able to follow up 85 of the original cohort of 98. The information showed that of these:

- 21% were deceased (not by suicide) with a mean age of death of 62 years;
- 22 remained in hospital (eight in units run by the same NHS Trust);
- Only ten were living in independent accommodation;
- Nearly 50% were in longer-term inpatient settings;
- Of those discharged, 50% were readmitted;
- Of the 67 who were alive at the time of follow-up, 54% were under a community mental health team, 27% were under an Assertive Outreach Team

(AOT) and 19% had no follow-up (four of whom were in placements outside of the city);

- There was a great deal of movement between units.

Whilst it may be appropriate for a minority of service users to remain in nursing care units for years, it is also important to ask whether such units are providing the most relevant and appropriately targeted interventions. Occupational therapy, which seeks to improve everyday living skills and engage people in valued activities, has traditionally been at the core of rehabilitation practice. However, a major study adopting precisely this focus failed to report any clinical advantage of a newly designed activity-based intervention over standard care (Killaspy et al., 2015).

One of the few studies to directly address problem behaviour in this group has been that by Leff and Szmidla (2002). They developed individually planned behavioural programmes supported by intensive psychological support and training for staff for "difficult to place patients". This programme was found to be effective in reducing violence and problematic social behaviour and removing barriers to resettlement into the community.

Anecdotally, we can say that where we have managed to establish SAFE as a service model, improved outcomes for service users with these complex mental health and behavioural needs can be observed. Over this period, we have managed to conduct a small number of studies examining various aspects of SAFE and will report on these where relevant throughout the book. However, the diverse nature of service provision for this group makes it difficult to carry out large-scale comparisons and relies on "practice-based evidence" (Meaden et al., 2015). With the increased drive to repatriate so-called out-of-area patients, and subsequent re-emphasis on commissioning services locally (Edwards et al., 2016), such larger-scale service evaluations may in the future become more viable.

In this book, we update and develop a number of the SAFE processes first described by Meaden and Hacker (2010), based on our experiences of the subsequent ten years. In particular, we have incorporated feedback from clinicians locally and nationally as well as made adjustments based on findings from research and service evaluation within the services we work in. This current book describes our most recent approach to meeting the needs of some of those with the most complex mental health and behavioural difficulties.

Chapter 1

Understanding Risk and Problematic Behaviour in Psychosis

Introduction

In focusing our intervention strategy primarily on risk and problematic behaviour reduction it is not our intention to focus exclusively on risk management to the exclusion of recovery values and principles. Behaviour change should never be the end goal but rather a step in the recovery process. However, problematic behaviour can be a significant barrier that prevents people from living independent meaningful lives. This, alongside poor engagement, is the main reason why people end up in long-term care settings. Distress is important too and is a strong motivator in help-seeking. Those who are distressed by their psychotic experiences may be easier to engage in treatments designed to reduce their distress. Conversely, those who report little distress and indeed may experience positive affect from their psychotic experiences (e.g. from appraising their voices intent as benevolent) or who view their problem behaviours as acceptable solutions to life's problems are likely to be harder to engage and present an increased risk (Meaden et al., 2012).

It is a common misperception, we would argue, that people are under the care of intensive psychiatric services due to enduring symptoms, that they are in some sense mentally ill or have intractable issues with substance misuse. The fact is that many people continue to have such problems but live in the community; perhaps not without significant problems, but people can and do experience symptoms of mental illness and nevertheless live well (Gibson et al., 2013) without professional support. What brings people into services is that they are distressed and therefore are help-seeking or they exhibit problem behaviour, which raises concern for themselves or others. It is true that these are seen in the context of mental health difficulties, but mental ill health is, in our view, not the primary reason for receiving care.

With this in mind, our aim is to tailor risk assessment and formulation to refocus care efforts and in keeping with UK national policy to reduce the potential impact of barriers to recovery and to nurture factors that assist it (Department of Health, 2007).

DOI: 10.4324/9781003082811-2

Risky or Challenging?

The Royal College of Psychiatrists (2007, p. 10) define challenging behaviour as

> When behaviour is of such an intensity, frequency or duration as to threaten the quality of life and/or the physical safety of the individual or others and is likely to lead to responses that are restrictive, aversive or result in exclusion.

The term challenging behaviour was first introduced by Blunden and Allen (1987) and was used within the learning disabilities population as a way for services to adapt the way they work to meet the needs of the service user rather than to use the term to describe an inherent problem with an individual. Emerson (2001) went on to describe how these behaviours refer to only behaviours which involve significant risks to others or serve to create access barriers to "community settings". He outlined three additional points when defining challenging behaviours:

1   Challenging behaviours are defined by their impact and the cause and topography will vary
2   Challenging behaviour is a social construct (what is defined as challenging may vary between setting and culture)
3   Challenging behaviour has wide-ranging personal and social consequences.

These broad ways of defining such behaviours well describe the territory of the behaviours we attempt to address in this book. They in effect encompass both risk (which primarily and objectively concerns harm) and challenging behaviour (which may be subjectively problematic and may indirectly lead to harm). However, for our purposes, it is more helpful to separate them as they can require different formulation and care planning processes. This enables us to be more focused on what we are addressing and be much clearer on our expected outcomes.

Paul Meehl's (1954) important historical delineation between clinical and actuarial (or statistical) approaches to risk assessment have been built on further by Douglas and Skeem (2005). The process of risk assessment exists on a continuum of rule-based structures, with completely unstructured approaches at one end of the continuum and actuarial assessment at the other end (Skeem & Monahan, 2011). The Structured Professional Judgment (SPJ) approach is the widely endorsed solution. However, SPJ does not go further and structure how the individual risk factors are to be combined in clinical practice (Skeem & Monahan, 2011). We may consider risk formulation as broadly the next stage of development with shared risk assessment the optimum method for drawing together all of the risk factors into a coherent picture. This constitutes our shared risk formulation template (see Chapters 3 and 4).

When dealing with more frequent, often daily, challenging behaviours we tend to find our Cognitive Approach to Risk Management (CARM) formulation more useful. This treats both static (e.g. past behaviour) and stable dynamic factors (e.g. command hallucinations) as vulnerability factors; helpful in understanding the function of problem behaviours but NOT the main focus of treatment. This is in contrast to the static-dynamic framework where dynamic stable factors would be part of the long-term treatment plan. CARM aims to address acute dynamic factors (the immediate precursors of the behaviour) and promote more adaptive responses to triggers, thus developing a coping repertoire. The likelihood of significant risk is often indicated by past offences that require a long-term plan and attempts to address factors associated with the risk at the time, which may or may not be present now. Efforts are typically made to test out the risk often by means of reducing restrictions (e.g. on leave). This monitoring and management can be effective but may limit the pursuit of recovery goals. Assessment and formulation of risk behaviours typically involve making estimates of the likelihood of the risk occurring. Often, it is accompanied by actuarial measures to support a process of making structured professional judgements. Our approach is to use the static-dynamic framework as described in detail in Chapter 4 which gives clear targets for long-term treatment and risk monitoring. These are intended to be idiosyncratic and therefore have high sensitivity and specificity as much as possible.

Risk behaviours in psychosis are well reported in the literature and are typically described as physical assault, use of weapons, damage to property (including arson), suicide (attempted and completed) and self-injury. We do not include sexual assault here since this is a specialist area in itself and arguably a less common feature of psychosis (see Meaden & Hacker, 2010 for a fuller discussion). By contrast, challenging behaviours have been far less researched and documented in relation to psychosis. These behaviours tend to be more frequent and the factors driving and maintaining them regularly present. This affords the opportunity to intervene in the here and now to pre-empt the behaviour and to enable the service user to develop more adaptive means of addressing the function in a more helpful way (e.g. being assertive when experiencing an unwanted intrusion from other service users instead of resorting to insults or making threats).

Among the few to write about challenging behaviour in people with psychosis have been Hogg and Hall (1992). They identified a number of common problematic behaviours in people with schizophrenia:

- Aggression (physical assaults on other people; damage to property; self-injury)
- Antisocial behaviour (shouting or screaming; swearing; spitting; recurrent and uncontrolled vomiting, smearing of faeces; stealing)
- Sexually inappropriate behaviour (nakedness in public; exposure of genitals; masturbation in public; sexual harassment/assault)
- Bizarre behaviour (stereotypic behaviour such as rocking or odd speech; using nonsense or jumbled words; unusual gait or hand movements; altered routine such as sleep reversal; unrestrained eating and drinking including dangerous substances

However, as with other attempts to capture and define problematic behaviours challenging behaviour and risk behaviour are mixed together.

More recently, Meaden and Hacker (2010) devised the Challenging Behaviour Checklist developed from staff surveys in the units we work across to capture the range of problem behaviours routinely encountered. We sought to categorise this list of 116 behaviours into 11 domains:

1 Intentionally/deliberate self-harm
2 Verbal aggression
3 Physical aggression against objects
4 Physical aggression towards others
5 Sexually inappropriate behaviours
6 Fire risk behaviours
7 Compulsive behaviours
8 Acquisitive behaviours
9 Absconding
10 Socially inappropriate behaviours
11 Behavioural deficits

As a checklist, it remains a useful tool in ensuring that we ask about all possible behaviour problems as well as enabling us to capture service-level and individual change (see Chapter 12). However, it is no longer our preferred assessment and formulation tool, as along with the early categories provided by Hogg and Hall (1992), it confounds challenging and risk behaviour.

Specific examples of what we now separately treat and define as challenging behaviours can include:

- Verbal aggression (making threats or insults, shouting, persistent screaming);
- Urinating in public;
- Smearing faeces;
- Spitting;
- Refusing requests;
- Lying on the floor (e.g. in the communal lounge);
- Regular regurgitation of food;
- Blocking exits;
- Entering the personal space of others;
- Over activity (repetitive pacing);
- Banging doors and window;
- Making frequent demands.

Whilst any of these behaviours may be less concerning than say assaulting another resident, if they are not appropriately addressed then not only can it have a significant direct impact on the service user (e.g. their leave being temporarily suspended; deterioration in physical and mental health), but it also impacts upon their carers (familial and professional) as well as other service users. Furthermore, it can negatively impact the service user's quality of life and can leave them to be subject to negative social responses such as inappropriate treatment, exclusion, abuse, deprivation and systematic neglect (Emerson, 2001). The Royal College of Psychiatrists (2007) helpfully suggest that it is the responsibility of staff and service providers to understand the origin and meaning of a person's behaviour and to establish what a person may be trying to communicate and for services to develop helpful ways to respond to these behaviours to better meet the service user's needs and reduce the challenging behaviour.

A common issue when working with staff and carers is in working with negative symptoms. Typically, these evoke unhelpful labelling such as "laziness". These behaviours are also regularly attributed to undesirable personality characteristics such as being "attention seeking" and can prove as frustrating to deal with risk behaviours such as assault. This requires a further way of categorising behaviours to socialise others away from implicitly ascribing a function to the behaviour and learning to simply describe the behaviour itself. In the previous SAFE work, Meaden and Hacker (2010) chose to categorise behaviours as excess or deficit behaviours presenting high or low risk. We have moved away from this labelling, partly as a means of adopting a more recovery-focused language and also in respect of the distinction between challenging and risk behaviours. The terms we have adopted are active and passive behaviours:

1   Active Behaviours

These constitute those where there is some form of motor activation whereby the individual physically initiates an action of some sort. This can be challenging for others (e.g. making racist remarks) or risk related (punching another resident in the face).

2   Passive Behaviours

These concern the absence of engaging in a behaviour. Again, these can be challenging (e.g. standing in front of a door and refusing to move) or risk related (e.g. not drinking for prolonged periods).

Some behaviours may appear as passive behaviours: lying on the floor. However, when their function is examined more carefully, they may in fact constitute active behaviours. These "active resistance behaviours" may serve as protests against unwanted rules, regulations and treatments (e.g. taking medication for diabetes, being asked to leave a communal area). These behaviours represent a clear motivation to engage in the behaviour. By contrast, those behaviours which are a result of an amotivational state are more clearly passive (e.g. lying in bed and lacking the motivation to get up).

Relationship Between Psychosis and Violence Risk: The Big 4

Many media portrayals have unhelpfully suggested that people hearing voices or having other psychotic experiences pose a significant threat. Whilst it is undoubtedly true that some people with psychosis act in dangerous ways or end their own lives, this is by no means the majority (Strode, 2017). In their study of 143 offenders with mental illness, Peterson et al. (2014) found that of the 429 offences committed by this population only 4% could be directly attributed to psychotic symptoms. When considering the risk behaviour in question, care should be taken to understand the relevant factors hypothesised to contribute to its occurrence. Put simply, people experiencing psychosis who act in dangerous ways do not necessarily do so as a function of their psychotic symptoms. Indeed, many risk assessment tools appear to tap into four much broader overlapping dimensions: criminal history, irresponsible lifestyle, psychopathy and criminal attitudes and substance abuse-related problems (Skeem & Monahan, 2011).

Despite a wealth of evidence to the contrary, historically, risk assessments of people with mental health difficulties continue to rely upon unstructured clinical opinion or the use of actuarial tools that statistically estimate the occurrence of risk (Hockenhull et al., 2012). This can lead to linking risk behaviours to the occurrence of psychotic experiences, for example acting on a command from a voice. In their review of 110 studies reporting on 45,533 individuals (18% of whom were violent) of risk factors for violence in persons affected by psychosis, Witt et al. (2013) identified a number of modifiable (dynamic) risk factors, including hostile behaviours, recent substance misuse, non-adherence to psychological therapies and poor impulse control. The most significant static factor was criminal history. Predicting future behaviour on the basis of past behaviour is a long-established experimental finding going back to the origins of the science of psychology (Thorndike, 1911). A past history of violent behaviour has consistently been shown to be predictive of violence in psychiatric groups and mentally disordered offenders (Andrews et al., 2006; Bonta et al., 1998) and remains the best predictor of future violence. An interesting 35-year longitudinal cohort study by Eriksson et al. (2011) highlights the importance of historical violence risk in some populations. These researchers were interested in predicting offending behaviour among individuals with no mental disorder by exploring the prevalence of risk factors for criminal offence reported at age 18 among males later diagnosed with schizophrenia. Also, they explored associations between risk factors reported at age 18 and lifetime criminal offence. The cohort studied involved 49,398 males conscripted into the Swedish Army between 1969 and 1970, of whom 377 were later diagnosed with schizophrenia. Strong associations were found between early misconduct, contact with the police or childcare authorities, crowded living conditions and arrest for public drinking. Having three of these four risk factors doubled the risk of offence among males with no later diagnosis of schizophrenia. The authors concluded that criminality in individuals with schizophrenia may at least partly be understood as a phenomenon similar to criminality in individuals in the general population. Clearly, this is a very specific cohort studied and so the findings may lack generalisability. Nevertheless, such studies point to those with psychosis as having a shared pathway to violence risk with other violent offenders.

A second key factor in understanding risk is the use of alcohol and other drugs which is universally agreed as being strongly associated with violence amongst the mentally disordered (Monahan et al., 2001; Swanson et al., 1990). Substance abuse increases risk by ten times (Monahan et al., 2001) and raises the risk regardless of diagnosis or symptoms. Reviewing 20 studies, Fazel et al. (2009) found that schizophrenia and other psychoses are associated with violence (particularly murder) but that most of the excess risk appears to be mediated by substance abuse.

A third important factor is personality disorder which is a strong predictor, especially if antisocial attitudes are evident (Monahan et al., 2001). Indeed, the presence of personality disorder features in most risk assessment scales (e.g. HCR-20). These factors require careful assessment and should not be just assumed from the negative effects that may be experienced when interacting with the person.

Fourthly, poor involvement in treatment represents a major feature of many risk scales which along with medication non-compliance has been strongly associated with future violence in psychiatric patients (Monahan et al., 2001; Swartz et al., 1998). However, those requiring rehabilitative interventions are likely to present in this way regardless of their risk. Care should therefore be taken to ensure that service users are not automatically categorised as being at higher risk simply because they refuse treatment.

To summarise, the main predicting factors are (1) past history; (2) substance use; (3) personality disorder; (4) poor involvement/engagement with treatment. These are more likely suspects than psychotic factors alone. Broader factors related to the person are varied and include symptom severity, history of violence, illness, age and antisocial attitudes (Blumenthal & Lavender, 2000; Quinsey et al., 2006). These encompass the Big 4, but the way in which symptom or illness severity may be relevant to understanding any given individual's risk requires careful assessment and formulation.

Cognitive-Behavioural Psychosis Risk Factors for Violence

Paranoid delusions have historically been associated with risk (Appelbaum et al., 2000) and in particular those where there is a perceived need to reduce threat or relieve distress (Swanson et al., 1996). These are often termed "threat control override symptoms" (TCO), which refers to the perception of threat which in reality does not exist or the belief that an outside entity is attempting to take control of one's mind. Rather than describe these as "symptoms", we would suggest that they constitute a specific type of belief that occurs in particular situations and is itself associated with heightened stress and anxiety. Regardless however of definition, TCO symptoms are associated with increasing the risk of violence twofold (Swanson et al., 1996).

Command hallucinations which command violence also appear to be important in understanding risk (Rogers, 2004, 2005), especially beliefs about voices (Trower et al., 2004; Birchwood et al., 2014). There is clear evidence now that beliefs about voices mediate both distress and behaviour and that the cognitive account of voices first proposed by Chadwick and Birchwood in 1994 (see Meaden et al., 2013 for a detailed account) is a valid model for understanding risk in relation to command hallucinations. Recent trial mediation analysis (Birchwood et al., 2017) has convincingly demonstrated that in relation to harmful behaviour the perceived power of voices to threaten and harm the individual or others relative to the perceived power of the individual to challenge and mitigate this threat (the power differential) is a strong predictor of compliance with hallucination commands. Further cognitive-behavioural factors deemed to be important in this mediation process include:

- Beliefs about the intent of the voice, with benevolence being more strongly associated with increased risk (Beck-Sander et al., 1997);
- Greater use of safety behaviours (Hacker et al., 2008) designed to avoid full compliance by partially complying or appeasing powerfully perceived voices;
- Generalised subordination to others and depression (Birchwood et al., 2004).

Clearly, psychotic symptoms play a role in risk behaviour. Understanding how beliefs about these symptoms mediate this risk is key to both formulating risk and identifying appropriate treatment targets.

Care Setting Factors in Violence Risk

Research on violence and aggression in inpatient settings suggests a role for external interpersonal factors such as overcrowding, management practices and staff inexperience (Whittington, 1994). This highlights the ongoing need for training, staff supervision and support. The likely target of aggression (staff versus other service users) appears to vary depending on the function of the behaviour. Aggression directed towards staff is more commonly associated with avoiding demands (forcing staff to acquiesce); rules being enforced or as a response to belittling interactional styles (Daffern et al., 2007).

Working with violence is a known risk factor for diminished mental health and turnover of staff. Interactions with violent service users have a serious impact on staff mental health and are associated with higher rates of psychological distress (Lamothe et al., 2021). One result is malignant alienation syndrome (Holmes, 2004), which describes how care relationships deteriorate and lead to a loss of sympathy and support from members of the team. Also commonly reported are cynicism and a sense of futility (Sambrook, 2008).

Cognitive-Behavioural Psychosis Risk Factors for Suicide

Rates of suicide vary considerably across studies ranging from 240 to 900 per 100,000 (Large & Ryan, 2014) compared to 12 per 100,000 globally across the general population (Varnik, 2012). People with schizophrenia (in particular males) who attempt suicide have a tendency to use more lethal means and consequently to have a higher likelihood of completion, with methods including jumping in front of traffic or trains, jumping off bridges, hanging or drowning (Powell et al., 2000; Shah & Ganesvaran, 1999).

Risk factors for suicide which apply to the general population also apply in schizophrenia. In their systematic literature review, Popovic et al. (2014) reported several risk factors implicated in suicide in schizophrenia. These were mainly related to affective symptoms (notably hopelessness independent of depression) alongside a history of suicide attempts and a number of psychiatric admissions. Other risk factors included younger age, closeness to illness onset, older age at illness onset, being male and evidence of substance abuse. As with violence risk, past history of suicide attempt increases the risk.

Research efforts have also focused upon trying to identify the period of highest risk for suicide. Links have been made to age with increased risk around the first episode or those in the early phases of their illness (Brown, 1997) and those over the age of 45 years (Hansen et al., 2004). Suicide risk also appears to increase following admission to acute psychiatric hospital or shortly following discharge (Pompili et al., 2007). Large and Ryan (2014) however caution against trying to identify high-risk groups as part of a risk assessment process. They argue that the assumption that those with schizophrenia belong to high-risk and low-risk groups and should therefore be managed differently on the basis of their risk status is deeply flawed. Simply being diagnosed with schizophrenia greatly multiplies a person's risk of suicide. It follows they suggest that it is neither possible to define a group who do not have an elevated absolute suicide risk when compared to the general community nor to define a high-risk group amongst those with schizophrenia who have an absolute risk of suicide at any given point. Thus, they go on to argue that the vast majority of the high-risk patients with schizophrenia will not progress to suicide. Whilst we routinely assess for suicide risk through our use of the START for this and other reasons, we strongly advocate careful formulation of individual risk behaviours.

Other Risks

Self-neglect behaviours which are commonly associated with psychosis (especially negative symptoms) are surprisingly less well researched; possibly because compared to violence or suicide they are less likely to be considered as important. Morgan (1998) is one of the few authors to have considered the issue of self-neglect in terms of risk and notes such problems are widespread in people with severe mental illness and extend beyond the scope of negative symptoms and tend to be judged as less serious. When considering the degree to which such behaviours present a risk and should be prioritised for intervention, it is useful to consider:

1   Whether self-neglect behaviours are in fact active resistance behaviours or arise as a result of an amotivational state
2   If neglect places the individual in a vulnerable position to others such that they may be exploited or abused (e.g. wearing dirty clothes, not washing, leaving their possessions in an unsafe place)
3   Whether the behaviour places the person at risk of physical health problems (e.g. malnutrition, risk of infection or disease)
4   Whether the behaviour leads to exclusion and isolation.

In one of the few studies in this area, Cowan et al. (2012) assessed the behaviour of 98 inpatients across ten 24-hour nursing care residential rehabilitation services using two measures: the Challenging Behaviour Checklist for Psychosis (CBC-P) (Meaden & Hacker, 2010) and the Resident Profile (Lelliott et al., 1996). They found that 17% were rated as having compulsive behaviours and 29% socially inappropriate behaviours potentially making them vulnerable to physical health problems, social exclusion or abuse and exploitation by others. All 98 had passive behaviours which could lead to social exclusion, result in abuse or exploitation by others as well as lead to physical health problems. Indeed, 36% were also rated as being at risk of developing a moderate-to-severe physical health problem.

The ABC of Risk: Refining the Cognitive Model

As noted earlier, particular beliefs seem to be important in mediating violence and other risks. However, whilst persecutory and voice-related beliefs may be present most of the time, individuals are not in an acute risk state at all times. In other words, people do not act on their beliefs at all times. Meaden and Hacker (2010) first proposed the role of specific beliefs triggered in specific situations in understanding the pathway to risk behaviours. The ABC formulation validated by Birchwood et al. (2017) provides a powerful tool for understanding distress and behaviour when applied to a specific situation.

Obtaining the B (Belief) proximally closest to the target behaviour is both crucial and revealing, demonstrating that it is not the delusional belief per se (i.e. the pan-situational belief present across many situations) that leads to the behaviour but, rather, it is the specific interpretation of a specific event; what we term the in-situation belief. Identifying these in-situation beliefs and the factors that contribute towards them is critical in addressing risk.

Case Example: Joey

Joey believes that there is a special team of CIA agents in the community who watch him, follow him and are waiting to kidnap him (a persistently present and distressing persecutory pan-situational belief). Mostly, he copes by avoiding busy crowds and leaves his house only in the early morning when he believes the agents are asleep (safety behaviours). Recently, he assaulted a man at a bus stop who was talking on his phone. He believed that this man was calling the agents. He "knew" this because he felt a tingling in his arm (actually an anxiety symptom). He had been feeling more stressed on this particular day following his watching of a news item on TV that morning about Russian spies. Joey punched the man in the face and ran away.

As can be seen, understanding Joey's risk behaviour is complex. Externally, it is not obvious why Joey punches the stranger in the face and runs away. Joey later reveals his appraisal (his in-situation belief) at the time:

> I just saw him there . . . got the feeling in my arm. That's a sign you know. For sure. Thought its best to hit him, slow him down from calling them.

These specific beliefs (related to the persecutory belief) are key to undertaking this risk behaviour but also the context of more distal stressors. In the past, Joey has attacked members of the public on a more regular basis. He has a history of substance use and has often been found to be intoxicated at the time, which lowers his inhibitions to act in a violent manner. In this example we can see how one of the Big 4 risk factors potentially interacts with Joey's belief system lowering the threshold for violence.

Viewing the situation in terms of an ABC formulation we can see in Table 1.1 the sequence and role of different types of belief.

Table 1.1 ABC Formulation

A (Activating event)	B (Belief)	C (Consequences – emotional and behavioural)
Watching TV report about spies before going on leave	*The CIA agents are out there watching me.* (Pan-situational belief) *I must be careful.*	Anxious Hypervigilant
Man at the bus stop talking and looking at me.	*He is one of the agents.* (In-situation belief 1)	Acute anxiety and somatic symptoms (Arm tingling)
(Arm tingling)	*It's a sign – he's about to call them.* (In-situation belief 2)	Anxious and feels threatened
Highly anxious and afraid	*Must stop him, slow him down.* (In-situation belief 3)	Hits man and runs away Relief that threat is reduced (Negative internal reinforcer)

Such ABC formulations are key in individual cognitive therapy work, but addressing them with harder-to-reach populations generally requires an integrative, multidisciplinary approach. For example colleagues who have an established relationship with less engaged service users (such as healthcare assistants, peer recovery workers or occupational therapists) can offer genuine insights from interactions that facilitate the development of hypotheses regarding the service users' inner world. Such hypotheses can be explored and clarified with service users through the process of Team Based Cognitive Therapy (TBCT) (see Chapter 8). In the following chapters, we proceed to describe each stage of the SAFE approach as we have developed it in collaboration with our multidisciplinary colleagues. We draw on research evidence, cognitive therapy, behavioural and forensic theory and our own theory–practice links in support of the principles we have adopted. The validity of SAFE we believe is best evidenced through case illustrations and specific recovery outcomes of the individuals with whom we work.

Summary

Understanding risk in those affected by psychosis requires an understanding not only of how psychotic symptoms and beliefs about them drive risk behaviours but also how factors such as personality and substance use contribute. Our refined cognitive model enables a more detailed appreciation of why individuals may experience persistent symptoms and hold relatively stable beliefs about them yet only exhibit risk behaviours under particular circumstances. The interplay between these complex factors can be seen more clearly through the lens of formulation and is best appreciated when it is shared.

Chapter 2

Getting Started

Assessing and Formulating the Team and the Service

Introduction

Getting innovations adopted into routine practice is often a slow process requiring careful, patient and persistent efforts, understanding the interpersonal dynamics and political context and local culture within which one is working, and how these may create potential barriers to change alongside identifying potential champions and allies. In this chapter, we share our experience of trying to introduce and implement SAFE. We reference the good practice literature and examine what lessons can be learnt from it and our own experiences.

Identifying Barriers to Change

When we first began to promote the use of SAFE beyond those services we directly worked in clinically, we became interested in research into strategies that might improve our chances of success. Greenhalgh et al. (2004) in a review of over 1,000 documents attempted to address the question: "how can we spread and sustain innovations in health service delivery and organization?" They found that innovations are more easily adopted if they:

1   Have a clear, observable, unambiguous advantage, such as greater effectiveness
2   Are compatible with the values, norms and perceived needs of the intended adopters
3   Are perceived by key players as simple to use
4   Allow intended users to experiment with them;
5   Can also adapt, refine or otherwise modify them to suit their own needs.

In our efforts to more clearly demonstrate the advantages of SAFE, we have evolved our framework further. SAFE as shown in the following chapters has adopted a more concise process and fits within and supports reflective practice. Perhaps more importantly, we now report (see Chapter 12) on our approach

DOI: 10.4324/9781003082811-3

to capturing change in the hard-to-reach population our work is primarily intended for.

The SAFE components we propose fit well with the increased priorities given to both risk assessment and management (Department of Health, 2007; The Royal College of Psychiatrists, 2007), whilst also supporting Multidisciplinary Team (MDT) assessment and care planning processes by improving communication (shared and documented understanding) and producing clear realistic care planning goals to better enable recovery. We emphasise understanding the person's own goals and reducing barriers to participation in ordinary community living. This is in keeping with the increased focus on recovery and promoting social inclusion in current mental healthcare (Keet et al., 2019).

Making SAFE simple and easy to use has been perhaps our greatest challenge. Inevitably, conducting detailed assessment, formulation and implementing consistent interventions on very specific behaviours is time-consuming and resource-intensive. Devising ways of streamlining SAFE has been a key objective. A significant step has been to combine Service Level Shared Formulation (SLF), CARM and static-dynamic formulation within a structured risk assessment process and incorporate all of these elements into reflective practice forums. This has enabled some inpatient services to complete all of these tools for all those in the service and review them regularly as part of routine clinical practice. It has been important in this process to experiment with and adapt SAFE, working closely with our MDT colleagues and as much as possible with our service users and their families. Experimenting with elements of the SAFE approach has been important and has fostered a collaborative spirit with MDT colleagues whereby we can examine which elements are most helpful in a given setting.

It is also useful to identify the most likely adopters. These tend to be those most motivated to use it by believing in its benefits and having the necessary skills to use it. They will also be more likely to adopt it if it meets a need that they have already identified. Where SAFE adoption has been successful, we have identified several key elements.

1   A fully staffed MDT including nursing, occupational therapy, psychology and psychiatry
2   A service philosophy focused on recovery
3   Clear aims and objectives for the service
4   A reliable service structure where meetings are relevant, well organised and planned (with clinically relevant information prepared in advance)
5   A culture where all contributions to clinical decision-making and discussion are encouraged and valued regardless of profession or grade
6   Involvement of the service user and carers in clinical discussions as much as possible
7   A commitment to timely and reliable completion of clinical and service assessments

Successful implementation is also more likely if the innovation has the same meaning for the services' senior management and other stakeholders (e.g. commissioners); for example, if everyone agrees that the innovation is likely to promote good quality risk assessment and care plans.

Assessing the Service

Services for those for whom SAFE is primarily developed may be broadly classified as rehabilitation services. Such services, and indeed the term itself, have declined significantly over recent years, with many of them closing down. However, rehabilitation is currently enjoying something of a renaissance in the UK, featuring as part of the ten-year Forward Plan (NHS, 2019) and the Getting it Right First Time initiative (NHS, 2019). Both acknowledge the need for specialist intensive MDT care for those with complex mental health and behavioural needs and are hard to reach and treat – precisely those for whom SAFE has been developed.

In order to better enable services to deliver rehabilitation interventions successfully, we have found it useful to help services look in detail at their processes and procedures. In our experience, service reviews have almost become a seemingly endless cycle. Typically, they focus on efficiency and cost issues and rarely on meaningful clinical outcomes: do they actually work? Moreover, we are interested in whether SAFE can help improve the service. Clifford et al. (1989) developed the QUARTZ system as a quality assurance process. The QUARTZ system originated in part from work by Lavender (1984, 1987), who aimed to develop a series of model standard questionnaires (Lavender et al., 1994), which would be flexible and collaborative. The intention was to facilitate service improvement within a hospital, through supporting change implementation and promoting a culture of ongoing service review. The tool itself involves a semi-structured interview focused across five areas.

1   Service aims
2   Referral, selection and admission
3   Programme planning and review
4   Case coordination and recording
5   Service review

We undertake QUARTZ reviews with key members of the MDT. Questions in each area relate to the delivery of predefined standards. At the conclusion of each QUARTZ area, summary ratings are made on a 4-point scale with descriptors pertaining to each point on the scale. We subsequently feed the results of the whole review back to the staff involved in the review process, making any amendments, including additional recommendations before feeding back the findings to all of the wider team. This is usually in the form of an away day aimed at generating possible solutions to any issues highlighted. Each area involves questions regarding a number of themes.

Service Aims

Identifying the client group for which the setting provides a service is an important first step. We try to understand what the service aims to achieve and how this is carried out. Asking about how the resources are allocated is a useful part of this process along with identifying what problems the service has with meeting its intended aims. The philosophy and values underlying the service provided are crucial to understand if these are shared by all staff and how in turn these are communicated to service users and their families.

For us, the aims of rehabilitation services should always address recovery barriers (e.g. problem behaviours) and promote engagement. We propose that alongside distress, these are the principal reasons why people come into rehabilitation services, and these constitute psychological factors rather than psychiatric ones (i.e. "symptoms").

Referral, Selection and Admission

Exploring where referrals come from and what is the process involved in making them are useful questions. In many of the services we work across, we strongly encourage the use of structured measures to ensure that those who are referred appropriately meet the service aims.

Importantly, QUARTZ asks if the setting has real control over who it admits. If inappropriate cases are accepted (often due to pressures and demands elsewhere within the care system or unclear referral and admission criteria), then the service will struggle to meet the needs of both these individuals and the core group for whom the service is intended. Those who have primarily personality-based problems often end up utilising a lot of staffing resources to the detriment of other service users experiencing psychosis. Staff must have the appropriate skills for working with particular needs (e.g. for those labelled with a personality disorder or autism spectrum disorder). For inpatient services, the physical setting must allow for appropriate opportunities for behavioural observation and for users to work on goals of independence (e.g. in cooking meals). In a community setting, those who present with frequent significant acute risks may pose too great a risk to be supported appropriately. Such cases may also overstretch the resources of the team, meaning that care cannot be adequately given to other users of the service.

Programme Planning and Review

Most settings operate some form of individualised care programme planning system, but it is useful to understand the rationale for it and what if any problems those using it experience. Eliciting what methods and tools (if any) are used to make an assessment on which to base care plans helps us to understand many aspects of how the service operates; most notably its commitment to evacuating objectively the care given. The scope of any assessment used is important in determining what areas of the user's life are generally considered in addition to understanding the person's clinical problems.

Examining who is involved in the care planning process and how they are involved (including the service user and their family) tells us a great deal about the collaborative nature of care and how (if at all) it reflects the aims and values of the service. Ideally, a clear need-adapted plan with defined responsibilities should be produced with overall goals translated into specific objectives or goals which are realistic and achievable. Critically, we should ask if all areas of the care plan are usually implemented or attempted and if they are regularly reviewed for success, with new plans devised to address the problems in a different way or build on any success. Discharge criteria are also important to understand. Indeed, service users can sometimes remain within a service for many years with no discernible benefit.

Case Coordination and Recording

Essentially, here we want to know who makes the decisions about service users' care and how collaborative this is. The quality of recording care and in particular incidents of problems are vital and, in our experience, are all too often incomplete, vague with key relevant information not easily accessible or shared. Often, inpatient services for such complex difficulties will have another case coordinator outside of the setting. How care is communicated and coordinated with such individuals is important to understand especially in regard to community activities, leave and discharge planning.

Service Review

In practice, this can take many forms but may not be carried out regularly. This is likely to store up problems, especially when the validity of the service is questioned. Ideally, the service should review itself annually including examining any data collected and analysing it in order to monitor, evaluate and review all aspects of the service. As part of this, we always ask whether the clinical outcomes of the service are being systematically measured and monitored.

Some areas however require more frequent timely review such as those involving serious incidents. It is important that there is sufficient opportunity for supportive non-critical debriefing with the opportunity to increase and utilise learning from the incident. These form part of our weekly reflective practice sessions on inpatient units.

Implications for SAFE

SAFE can help teams and those who use the service with problems identified across all of these five areas of the QUARTZ system. Typically, we find that services are unclear about their remit both in terms of their role within the local care pathway and their service aims. If all staff do not share common aims and a shared purpose, then care is likely to become fragmented. Consequently, contradictory messages and expectations are likely to be communicated to those who use the service or refer to it.

Often, there is a lack of rigour and consistency with regard to the gathering and use of information about engagement and risk issues. This is particularly important as staff can become easily frustrated when those admitted or taken under the care of the team do not meet staff expectations or skill sets. The ability of a given service to tolerate disruption and manage risk is key to aiding recovery and avoiding placement breakdown. In their international Delphi study, Turton et al. (2010) aimed to identify specific factors of care that key stakeholders regarded as most important in promoting recovery for people with longer-term mental health problems in institutional care. One of the most important domains to emerge was staff attitudes. This domain included building good therapeutic alliances characterised by qualities of communication and interaction that were polite, honest, equal, attentive, respectful, accepting and understanding.

Many services we have encountered lack a systematic assessment process, the adoption of which is vital to assess both appropriate referrals and evaluate progress and change. Few services carry out an annual review and examine their outcome data; utilising this to reflect upon the effectiveness of the service and identify areas for improvement. Ideally, services are open to change and willing to explore the benefits of adopting new approaches such as SAFE. There of course are a variety of care approaches available in addition to SAFE, but we would argue none to our knowledge provides a coherent MDT-based framework targeted at addressing problem behaviour in those who are hard to reach and treat.

Formulating the Team

Some attempts have been made to examine the broader process and impact of team formulation (see also Chapter 3) and identify service development opportunities. Taylor and Sambrook (2012), for example, explored the value of a cognitive interpersonal model in formulating key staff–service user relationships and whether such an approach would yield useful team-based interventions in an inpatient setting. They found that this type of team formulation was indeed effective in making sense of interactions contributing to the maintenance of service users' challenging behaviours and staff burnout and assisted in developing systemic interventions likely to effect change and guide service development planning. Short et al. (2019) explored definitions applied to team formulation and the interrelationship between the team and the process of formulation, utilising convergent qualitative synthesis design and thematic analysis to transform evidence from quantitative and qualitative studies into qualitative findings. Emergent themes were having "increased knowledge and understanding", "altered perceptions, leading to altered relationships, feelings and behaviours", "space to reflect", "useful when stuck or challenged", "perceived increase in effectiveness" and "improved team working".

Whilst such research has been useful in understanding the merits of team formulation as applied to clinical problems and helping the team improve, attention has not been paid to the potential benefits of formulating the team as a whole. All clinicians will likely make idiosyncratic formulations (albeit informally) at some point about the team they work in and the services in which they work. However, it is considerably preferable to undertake this as an explicit and shared process. This will depend upon a number of factors. Very established team cultures can be hard to penetrate and change. We have encountered several where teams stick closely to the way they have always worked and heavily resist the introduction of any new approaches. In a number of cases, this has led to service closure since they have often been viewed externally as functioning poorly and unable to change or adapt. Time needs to be taken in these cases, learning patiently to understand the reasons for the established way of working along with who the key players and potential allies are.

Chaotic services are equally tricky, such as those where individual clinicians operate independently. There may be no "I" in team, but there are four in multidisciplinary! Simply locating a number of individuals in a building or shared office space does not make them a team. Remote working and hot desking may add to any fragmentation, especially in community settings.

Meaden et al. (2015) have pointed to the strong parallels that exist between service user's engagement and treatment and the engagement of the team and their receptivity to new approaches. Often, we have encountered (especially those involved in rehabilitation services) teams which have been neglected, with clinicians all but burnt-out and alienated from service users and their needs. To start to understand teams, including those that may be operating in a dysfunctional manner, useful team formulation questions include the following.

- What do team members identify as being the main problems they face?
- What has led to these problems? The history of the team may be usefully considered here along with what challenges they have faced.
- Where do the team and their members locate the problems they experience: where does the attribution (bias) lie?
- What are the pan-situational care beliefs of members of the team?
- What maintains the problems?
- What attempts have been made thus far to solve them?
- Have these worked at all?
- Is there a culture of learnt helplessness or hopelessness?
- What strengths does the team have?

These can be explored gradually and sensitively as the relationship with the team grows. Service or team "away days" can provide a useful, more explicit opportunity to explore the team's functioning, albeit couching questions carefully. Christofides et al. (2012) have described how informal team formulation can be implemented flexibly through an array of interactions with team members.

Obviously, some team members may be reluctant to share their views whilst others will be unlikely to disclose negative views. Reflective practice, once established as a safe place, can be a useful space to explore beliefs and attitudes. Murphy et al. (2013) and Wilcox (2013) have all reported on using reflective practice in the context of consultancy with team-level difficulties (e.g. "splitting"), when the work with service users was the focus of reflections. We now incorporate our risk assessment and formulation processes into reflective practice sessions with teams. Focusing on problem behaviours provides a useful catalyst for the discussion of staff's beliefs, attitudes and care behaviours.

Self-disclosure by the SAFE clinician can also be helpful. We often freely acknowledge our own biases and thoughts, along with how we have reflected on these. These processes are similar to those that many clinicians will be familiar with in individual therapeutic relationships. Care needs to be taken to build trust, empathy, and acknowledge the challenge and frustrations of the work without judging those we work with.

Exploiting Introductory Opportunities

The assessment areas drawn from Clifford et al. (1989), together with a formulation of the team, provide a rich amount of information to enable the SAFE clinician to decide where initial efforts may be best made. The SAFE clinician's role in the organisation will also influence the opportunities they have to draw on support from more senior management and lead clinicians in effecting change. SAFE can provide solutions to problems in any of the five areas drawn from Clifford et al. (1989). Just as we would socialise service users into a therapy model when engaging in individual therapy, so we are often socialising clinicians and teams into the SAFE approach.

Assessment and Outcome Tools

Our original and predominantly ongoing focus in SAFE has been on services best described as rehabilitation, both inpatient and in the community. Rehabilitation itself has been described as an "evidence free zone" (Killaspy, et al., 2005), and this has been associated with service closures and increased scrutiny of the effectiveness of such specialist teams. Disappointingly, evidence of positive outcomes from studies of specialist rehabilitation and AOTs has not emerged (e.g. Killaspy et al., 2006). This, we propose, is due to the correct outcomes not being effectively measured. If we accept that distress and behaviour along with poor engagement are the principal reasons for accessing mental health services, and poor engagement with services and treatment a key factor in detention, then these become the main areas we should be measuring. Service reviews have often led us to identify either the complete absence of service user and service-related outcome measures or the use of measures which consistently yield disappointing results. The introduction of tools such as the CBC-P (Meaden & Hacker, 2010) and the Residential

Rehabilitation Engagement Scale (RRES) for psychosis (Meaden et al., 2012) has been helpful in informing both evaluation of the service and care planning. Whatever clinicians may view as the reasons for service users receiving care, these tools help to focus attention towards SAFE intervention targets: the problem behaviours which act as barriers to recovery.

Service Evaluation and Review

As noted earlier, reviewing, auditing and evaluating services have almost become a continuous cycle. Schemes such as AIMS accreditation (Royal College of Psychiatrists, 2007) have been specifically developed with rehabilitation services in mind. However, whilst helpful in providing some quality assurance, AIMS is somewhat broad in its objectives and may be less helpful in examining the fundamentals of teamworking and ensuring fidelity to a clinical model. Conversely, the Dartmouth Assertive Community Treatment Scale (DACTS) developed by Teague et al. (1998) assesses model fidelity but also does not fully examine MDT functioning outside of this. More generally, service review and audit often focus on productivity with a strong focus on costs and funding. We have found that despite being developed some years ago, the QUARTZ system (Clifford et al., 1989) summarised earlier is still surprisingly relevant in terms of its focus on service users and carers and understanding team processes. We have used this to good effect, often feeding the findings back in a team "away day" offering a non-judgemental approach and emphasising team problem-solving. These have proven a good platform for introducing SAFE assessment tools and formulation processes.

Reflective Practice and Shared Formulation

Whilst there is somewhat mixed evidence regarding the impact of formulation in its various forms, overall, the consensus is that it can have a number of direct and indirect benefits (see Chapter 3). Team formulations enable broader knowledge and a deeper understanding of service users as well as providing a space to discuss cases and improve clinical practice (McTiernan et al., 2021). They help the team to improve their clinical care by utilising psychological theory and the person's experiences (Butler, 2006). Formulation can also be seen to have wider impacts on the team. Inpatient settings in particular can experience significant barriers to team efficiency due to low staffing levels and shift patterns (Robson & Quayle, 2009). Formulation has been found to increase team efficiency (Lake, 2008) and decrease feelings of frustration (Robson & Quayle, 2009).

Murphy et al. (2013) explored perceptions of what they termed "psychological consultation" on staff working in older adult inpatient services. They examined its impact on daily practice and the mechanisms of change involved using qualitative thematic analysis. They found that formulation consultation sessions improved team cohesiveness and effectiveness as well as the mental health of the team. It also appeared to increase psychological thinking about clients' presentations and enabled the development of care plans with greater emphasis on achieving successful discharge. Emergent themes suggested that psychological consultation enabled staff to better understand clients within the context of their lives, leading to improved relationships and more supportive care. Such formulation sessions appeared to impact on staffs' practice most when it focussed on especially complex presentations. Indeed, arguably, teams are most motivated to engage in shared formulations by what frustrates, upsets or even scares and intimidates them – just like service users.

A useful place to start then is often with the most complex cases that staff struggle most with. Offering the right type of formulation will be important. Risk formulation can convey the message that the SAFE clinician is taking team concerns seriously as well as providing a more detailed understanding of the risk and contributing to clear guidance on how best to manage it.

The SAFE Service Level Formulation taps into the strengths identified by Murphy et al. (2013) by helping the service to review their clinical aims and objectives. Very often, we have encountered services where service aims have drifted, with a lack of clear direction for service user's needs, over-attention to clinical recovery (such as alleviation of symptoms) and a neglect of personal recovery, which can lead to frustration amongst the team and service users alike. Focusing on recovery goals for the service user and barriers to these has helped enable the team to be much clearer and more realistic on the way forward. We now use this regularly when reviewing service user's needs and also capturing often small but personally meaningful change (see Chapter 12 for a detailed description). Berry et al. (2009, 2015) have also presented team formulation as a service-level intervention to help staff develop skills, confidence and effective relationships with service users.

The extent to which existing formulation models are appropriate to addressing the specific problems identified should also be considered. One of our qualitative explorations of how teams use and perceive the benefits of adopting a broad person-level formulation (the 5 Ps) for the purpose of understanding risk (Lynch, 2014) found that whilst they served a useful information-sharing function, there appeared to be little emphasis on developing positive risk-taking, with the focus more towards defensive practice. Additionally, not all staff saw a clear value or advantage of the approach. Neither was it viewed as being entirely compatible with the team's values and norms. Formulation models such as the 5Ps tend to collapse all of the person's problems together, such that it is difficult to accurately differentiate and hypothesise which factors lead to which problems. This can be confusing for the team and will not lead readily to clearly targeted interventions to address risk or problem behaviour.

"Reflective practice" is an imprecise concept which, in practice, may cover a range of broadly related activities. We have focused our work around facilitating a team's ability to reflect collectively upon team objectives, practices and processes, sharing information and understanding outcomes. The aim of reflective practice in SAFE is therefore to build shared understandings and support the work of the team. In our clinical practice, we have noticed an increasing number of services, keen to offer some form of reflective practice or team supervision as a means of promoting a more compassionate work culture and improving teamworking. We have utilised these opportunities to promote SAFE by linking together a number of components:

1   Completing structured risk assessment as a team
2   Developing SLFs;
3   Reflecting on, identifying and celebrating service user improvements;
4   Challenging assumptions and negative attitudes regarding service users and their behaviours;
5   Providing a supportive space to reflect on work with especially difficult episodes of care.

Training

Training presents an ideal opportunity to both increase skills and weave in clarification of SAFE concepts. Depending on the training requirements of a given team, we have found the following range of workshops to be helpful in promoting the use of SAFE:

1   Using and understanding assessment tools (using the CBC-P and our Recovery Goal Planning Interview, [Meaden & Hacker, 2010], the RRES for psychosis, [Meaden et al., 2012])
2   Understanding risk and challenging behaviour (models of risk, the CARM formulation, Early Warning Signs of Risk)
3   Basics of cognitive therapy (understanding the ABC model, relocating the problem from the A to the BC)
4   Rediscovering behavioural interventions (learning theory basics, applying reinforcement principles within a recovery framework, using Positive Behaviour Support plans).

When further embedded within reflective practice/team formulation sessions, this training can be consolidated into routine clinical practice.

Summary

We have discussed in this chapter how SAFE can be introduced along with some of the potential benefits. However, SAFE does have its limitations. Not all services and teams will be receptive or they may have their own models which are preferred and already embedded. Nonetheless, we hope that some elements of

SAFE will still prove useful. We would maintain that our different levels and types of formulation remain valuable and are greatly preferable to a single formulation approach. One size or type of formulation does not fit all. Measuring the right outcomes (see also Chapter 12) also remains for us relevant to all services, and we again emphasise that it is distress and problem behaviours that bring people to mental health services and as such, these should be the focus.

Chapter 3

Shared Formulation
Principles and Practice in SAFE

Introduction

Formulation is central to the work of SAFE – it's even in the name! SAFE formulations are used by the service to develop an understanding of the service users' needs and difficulties in order to support them in recovering a life that they find meaningful and satisfying. In order to effectively describe the principles and practice of SAFE, it is necessary to define what we mean by formulation and describe how this is conducted with teams as part of the SAFE approach. This chapter introduces the main SAFE formulations used throughout this book and explains how these are used with the team.

What Is Formulation?

Psychological formulation can be defined as a set of hypotheses about a person's difficulties, usually covering possible causes and maintaining factors (Eells, 2007). Formulation provides a way of organising and making sense of the different factors that are hypothesised to contribute to a person's problems and are at their best when they involve the service user in the sense-making process (Johnstone, 2018). Different psychotherapeutic approaches have different ways of formulating, and usually the formulation is taken to be grounded in psychological evidence of some kind (i.e. a theoretical model or research evidence that supports the presence of the factors within the formulation). While some formulations are very structured (such as those in SAFE), others are organised more like a narrative, describing the service user's experiences, the meanings attached to these and the possible psychological processes that maintain them. Ultimately, the goal of formulation is to make sense of the person's difficulties and provide ideas about possible intervention plans (Johnstone, 2018). A more recent development is that of team formulations. Team formulation has been described as a process through which a group of professionals develops a shared understanding of a particular clinical problem or difficulty experienced by a service user (Johnstone, 2018). Team formulation has been positioned as central to the role of clinical psychologists, particularly as a component of team leadership (Skinner & Toogood, 2010).

DOI: 10.4324/9781003082811-4

Team formulations, such as those in SAFE, are used to help the MDT to have a coherent view of the service users' needs and involve the team in coherent interventions guided by the shared formulation.

Formulations: The Evidence

Although formulation is a popular notion that is supported in the UK by the Division of Clinical Psychology (DCP) of the British Psychological Society (DCP, 2011), the evidence for psychological formulation having a positive impact on therapy outcomes is not strong (Bieling & Kuyken, 2003; Kuyken, 2006). One of the difficulties of measuring the impact of formulation is the range of definitions and approaches, and this applies to team formulations also. In a recent systematic review of the area, Geach et al. (2018) found a myriad of different definitions and descriptions of team formulation and summarised these as overlapping types variously including reflective practice meetings, sharing ideas informally and formulation-focussed consultation. All were unified by the core aim of developing a shared understanding (Geach et al., 2018). The review identified some modest outcomes possibly linked to team formulation, such as improved staff attitudes and ward atmosphere (Geach et al., 2018). However, due to the form that team formulations can often take (e.g. sharing ideas informally), the studies that have explored team formulation impact on outcomes are usually poorly controlled and so any observed changes (e.g. ward atmosphere) cannot be attributed with confidence to the implementation of team formulation due to the many potential confounding factors.

Short et al. (2019) conducted a systematic qualitative review that aimed to synthesise the results of a range of studies exploring team formulation, with an emphasis on the team processes of shared formulation. Similar to Geach et al. (2018), they found inconsistent definitions and a range of different ways of conducting psychological team formulations. While no studies were found that explored how the team influenced the formulation, the general findings suggested the team were affected by the formulation in a variety of ways. These included "increased knowledge and understanding", "altered perceptions, leading to altered relationships, feelings and behaviours", "space to reflect", "useful when stuck or challenged", "perceived increase in effectiveness" and "improved team working" (Short et al., 2019, p. 20). It is unclear to what extent these effects on the team translate into changes for service users, but this demonstrates some evidence that formulations are at least perceived by teams to be useful.

It is perhaps unsurprising, if somewhat disappointing, that evidence for team formulation is weak, given the fuzzy definitions and multiple ways of operationalising the process of conducting a team formulation. Furthermore, the goal of formulation – developing a shared understanding – is an outcome in itself, and so the ways in which the effects of a formulation are measured need to be closely aligned to this function. In SAFE, there is a clear rationale for the role of team formulation in serving a coordinating function that mobilises the resources of the team in an attempt to understand the experiences and problems of the service user. It is also a process through which other functions can be achieved, such as TBCT that targets unhelpful staff attributions. Each formulation in SAFE serves a different purpose and can be deployed in a strategic manner to achieve the goals of the service in enabling the recovery of the service user. However, given the generally weak evidence for team formulation in generating clinical change, we should remain open to testing and revising the hypotheses generated through the SAFE approach and regarding the approach itself. Research into the effectiveness of the approach is ongoing and we discuss this further in Chapter 12.

Shared Formulation in SAFE

Shared formulation is a core component of SAFE, and this is well described in the original text (Meaden & Hacker, 2010). As with any approach, SAFE is evolving and being refined based on our work and feedback from service users and colleagues. This section describes how shared team formulations are understood in SAFE, the processes through which they are deemed to be helpful and the expected outcomes associated with them.

Within SAFE there are a range of formulations, and these are designed to develop an understanding of the various psychological factors that contribute to the service user's difficulties. They draw on a range of psychological theories and evidence relevant to people who experience complex and enduring psychosis and have behavioural needs. Overall, the formulations are perhaps best described as being derived from cognitive behavioural traditions, informed by the recovery movement (Anthony, 1993). With the exception of the SLF, all the formulations focus on understanding the nature of the distress and problematic behaviour associated with psychosis, based on the core principles of cognitive therapy for psychosis (Birchwood & Trower, 2006). The function of a shared formulation is for the clinical team – that is all of those involved in the care of the service user – to develop a shared understanding of the key difficulties the service user faces that may impede their recovery and detract from quality of life and well-being, along with the different factors that contribute to the presentation and maintenance of these. As each formulation has a different intended outcome, we shall visit each in turn to discuss how it achieves its function. Blank templates of these shared formulations can be found in Appendices 1–4.

The Service Level Formulation

This formulation is designed to help the team understand the different factors that might be contributing to the person's need to be in services. It aims to answer the question: why can't the person leave our service right now? This formulation aims to identify barriers to the person's recovery and can be broadly conceptualised as those that are located at the level of symptoms and disabilities, internal barriers, external barriers and social participation (having a meaningful presence in their valued community, i.e. attaining valued social roles or functions) which the person is prevented from engaging in (see Appendix 1).

We have found it helpful to view symptoms of mental and physical illness similar to disabilities. In the primary target group of SAFE, these are all ongoing problems which may limit the person's ability to live an independent socially inclusive life. They include persistent distressing voices, persecutory delusions, cognitive deficits as well as diabetes, heart disease and respiratory disorders. However, as with those who have a disability or a long-term illness in the general population, with appropriate adaptations and support they can lead a meaningful valued life.

What prevents the person from achieving their important roles and goals are internal and external barriers. Internal barriers are those imposed by the person. They may not be readily aware of these or able to easily change them, and they may impose them for good reasons, but they nevertheless function as barriers. They include negative or antisocial attitudes, problem behaviours, unhelpful emotional reactions, poor frustration tolerance, poor engagement, denial of difficulties and symptoms/disabilities. External barriers are those imposed from outside of the person. These may be specific to the setting such as restricted leave, being detained under the Mental Health Act or external to the setting, such as lack of social contacts, absent family.

The SLF is useful in helping to crystallise the team's understanding of the key problems faced by the service user and agree areas to be focussed on for care planning. It is also useful in helping to map out the range of difficulties faced by the service user, and as such can also be used as part of ongoing outcome measurement (which will be discussed in Chapter 12). This formulation does not, however, attempt to explain why each factor identified is a problem for the person, abstaining from speculating on aetiological or maintenance factors. Instead, it maps out some of the areas of need, so that these can be formulated further using the other formulation structures.

The Cross-Sectional Formulation

This is often referred to as the "ABC" formulation. Its purpose is to develop an understanding of the cognitive and behavioural mechanisms that may be mediating distress and problematic behaviour. This is particularly useful in starting to develop empathy amongst the team and instil a sense of curiosity towards the service user's difficulties and needs. Also, it can be viewed as a precursor to the CARM formulation, which is a more structured and detailed blend of the cross-sectional formulation, behavioural formulation and functional analysis. The cross-sectional formulation is derived from traditional cognitive therapy theory, particularly rational emotive behaviour therapy (Ellis, 2004) and based primarily on the work of Paul Chadwick, Peter Trower and Max Birchwood (Birchwood & Trower, 2006; Chadwick et al., 1996). Underpinning this model is the notion that it is not events themselves that are distressing – including psychotic

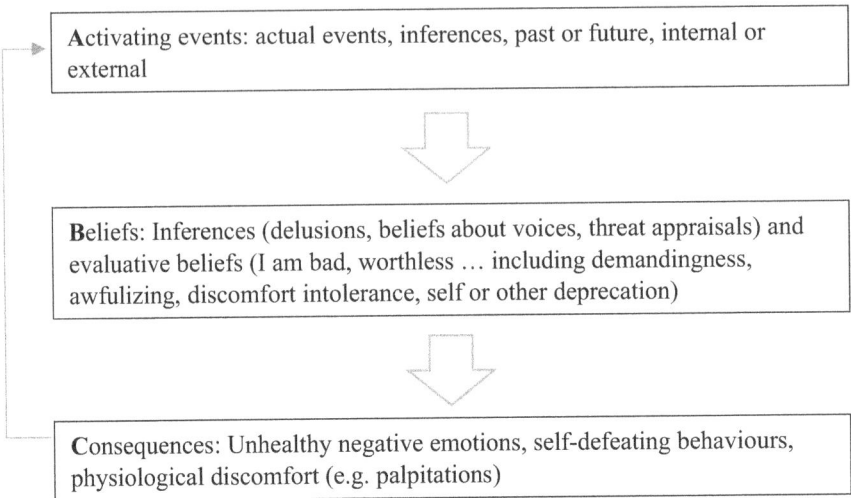

Figure 3.1 The Cognitive ABC Formulation

phenomena – but the meanings and appraisals assigned to them by the service user. Focus shifts away from symptoms (A) to the meanings of these for the person (B) and the emotional and behavioural consequences of these (C). A useful summary is provided by Bennett and Pearson (2015), and this is adapted in Figure 3.1.

It is helpful to clarify that for ease of use, the ABC components are considered in a linear, sequential fashion but that this should not be taken to assume that causality flows in a linear sequential fashion and that C can affect A and B, as well as B can affect A. Typically, the C is the behaviour or emotion that staff (and/or service user) are struggling with and this is clarified first with A, followed by B. It should go without saying that it requires detailed knowledge of the service user and discussion with them to be able to populate section B accurately, as they are the only ones who have access to their internal world and meaning-making.

The Cognitive Approach to Risk Management Formulation

CARM may stand on its own as a way of understanding and developing interventions for high-frequency behavioural excesses (Meaden et al., 2015) or behavioural deficits (Fox & Meaden, 2015). We have recently incorporated the CARM formulation into our wider risk assessment framework, which it now supports as a core model for formulating how factors identified through structured clinical judgement schemes such as the Short Term Assessment of Risk and Treatability (START; Webster et al., 2004) contribute to identified behavioural risks. This particular aspect will be discussed further in Chapter 4.

The overall structure of a CARM formulation can be seen in Appendices 2 and 3. CARM is based on functional analytic theory and starts with a clearly and operationally defined problematic behaviour. It is critical here to move away from poorly defined and fuzzy descriptions of behaviour that imply a function (such as "manipulating others"). Vulnerability factors capture the psychological dispositions, personality factors, developmental factors, functional impairments and other enduring aspects of the person. These also include pan-situational beliefs associated with psychotic symptoms (e.g. the world is dangerous). Setting events can be considered as exacerbations of the vulnerability factors that make the target behaviour more likely to occur. Although still distal in time from the occurrence of the behaviour, they represent a build-up in the motivational state towards action. Setting events may be external (e.g. having an argument) or internal (e.g. persistent derogatory voices). Early Warning Signs of Risk (EWS-R) are the observable signs of the internal setting events alongside the external setting events and can be a useful component of risk management planning. Triggers are events that lead (almost) immediately to the target behaviour, and these can be external (e.g. an insult from another) or internal (e.g. a voice command, anger). The last component of CARM is the reinforcers – events that follow the behaviour and maintain it or make it more likely to occur again in future. Positive reinforcers involve a consequence being added as a result of the behaviour (e.g. gaining care from others), while negative reinforcers involve the removal of something as a result of the behaviour (e.g. voices quieten down). Again, these can be external (e.g. breaking a window to avoid being discharged; negative reinforcement) or internal (e.g. intimidating other service users to feel powerful; positive reinforcement).

In staff training, we often use a metaphor to understand the steps of CARM, imagining that the problematic behaviour is the fire we wish to control. Here, the vulnerability factors are the combustible fuel; the setting events are the heat that creates the necessary conditions; the trigger is the spark that ignites the fire; the reinforcers are the oxygen that keep the behaviour going.

The Static-Dynamic Shared Risk Formulation

It is perhaps the risk formulation that has been refined the most substantially since the previous publication of SAFE (Meaden & Hacker, 2010). The current conceptualisation retains the distinction between static, dynamic stable and dynamic acute factors, but it recognises that results from assessment of these can usefully be incorporated into other formulation structures that propose clear functional links between the different levels, mostly the CARM formulation. We retain the structure usefully defined by Ward and Beech (2004) and conceptualise risk factors as static (immutable, unchangeable factors that generally increase risk of the target behaviour reoccurring), dynamic stable (slowly changing factors) or dynamic acute (rapidly changing factors that often directly precede a high-risk event). In our regular work with service users and teams within inpatient psychiatric rehabilitation units, we use a variety of risk assessments such as the START (Webster et al., 2004) or the HCR-20 (Douglas et al., 2013) to support the identification of risk factors. Once identified as relevant for a particular risk behaviour, the factors can be understood across the three areas and incorporated into a formulation that describes how the factors identified in the risk assessment, alongside other more general psychological factors, function to influence risk. In effect, we are answering the question: under what circumstances would the risk event (problematic behaviour) be likely to be observed? Key to this is having a clearly defined and operationalised risk behaviour identified, and each problematic behaviour often requires a separate formulation to understand the contributing factors. We describe the incorporation of this and the CARM formulation in more detail in Chapter 4.

Implementation of SAFE Formulations

All of our shared formulations can be completed in isolation or as part of a comprehensive process for understanding a service user's needs, planning and evaluating their care. All are best completed by the full range of disciplines representative of the whole MDT. This helps to ensure that there is the full range of perspectives as well as promoting buy-in from all members of the team. Formulations are also much more comprehensive and holistic when they include the perspectives of service users and family members. Unfortunately, it is easy to find teams operating in-group and out-group processes when all disciplines are not represented within the formulation team. In our experience it is most common to be missing representatives from the medical team, which can be particularly problematic when discussing risk formulations and barriers to recovery such as leave arrangements that they have the ultimate clinical responsibility for reviewing. As such, we strongly advocate for a whole team approach to shared formulation, particularly when implementing SAFE at a service level.

Understanding Why Service Users Are in the Service

If implementing SAFE as a service approach, we generally recommend commencing the process with the SLF. This allows for the development of a shared appreciation of the needs of the service user, identifying potential treatment targets to enhance independence and supporting effective care planning. The SLF is often helpful when as a team we are unsure what we are doing or why a service user is placed with us: it helps to clarify their needs and crystallise the team's thinking about the ways of understanding possible approaches towards them. The SLF by its nature is quite descriptive, and as such functions as a snapshot or map of the barriers to recovery for the service user at a particular time. Because of this, we have found it useful to reformulate the SLF annually, reviewing the different factors and updating them:

- No change: black font
- Deterioration: red font

- Improvement: green font
- Maintained improvement (at 3rd SLF): blue font
- Barrier overcome: strike-through font

This simple methodology allows us to both monitor change over time and reinforce the efforts of care staff in reflective practice and the service user and their carers at care planning meetings. Our experience suggests that the wider MDT finds this use of the tool effective at identifying meaningful change in difficulties that otherwise do not seem to be captured by traditional outcome metrics (see Chapter 12).

Appreciating Idiosyncratic Meaning and Developing Empathy

Cognitive therapy ABC formulations can be a useful starting point for maintaining team curiosity and helping to develop empathy towards the service user. Since meanings and beliefs cannot be fully realised without the involvement of the service user, this is a useful starting point for integrating their views and contribution to the process of assessment and formulation. Members of the team who have a better relationship with the service user can be supported to try to engage them in the process of formulation. Trigger events that appear significant to the team may not be to the service user, and equally, seemingly innocuous events from the team's point of view may have particular significance for the service user. It is imperative to explore these and the different meanings of the events. Once the meanings, appraisals and attributions have been explored, ways of modifying these can be discussed, either through TBCT (see Chapter 8) or through one-to-one therapy, if the service user is able and willing to engage in this. Alternatively, the details of the formulation can be used to seed the development of a CARM template. We have found the ABC formulations particularly helpful when starting to think about high-frequency challenging or risk behaviours that teams find problematic. This deceptively simple cornerstone of cognitive therapy begins the process of considering internal cognitive processes such as idiosyncratic appraisals and interpretations of events. This then starts the work of developing the team's awareness of the importance of the service user's meaning-making, setting the stage for TBCT of unhelpful attitudes held by members of the team and paving the way for the later introduction of CARM or static-dynamic risk formulation (as appropriate), which requires an increasingly sophisticated consideration of the service users' point of view.

Towards the Understanding and Management of Problematic Behaviour

Typically, CARM formulations are best used for high-frequency active challenging behaviours, such as verbal and physical aggression towards others. These are relatively easy to operationalise and define, and the teams are usually quite motivated to try to manage these, perceiving the intrinsic value in generating EWS-R for this purpose. Our team supervision sessions are the format we now adopt for bringing together the various disciplines for gathering the information required for a CARM formulation. Healthcare assistants, technical assistants and assistant psychologists are particularly useful here as they tend to have more daily contact with service users. Prior to meeting, it is helpful if a thorough review of the service user's clinical notes is carried out (the Personal, Social and Psychiatric History Interview is especially helpful here, see Meaden & Hacker, 2010). It is rare that a CARM formulation can be completed in one sitting, and so various roles for further assessment and information gathering can be identified and shared between sessions to support the next meeting.

We have moreover adapted the CARM formulation for "passive behaviours" (previously termed behavioural deficits or negative symptoms; Fox & Meaden, 2015); however, these are more difficult to formulate, as the behaviour itself is often problematic due to its absence (e.g. self-neglect), external reinforcers may be absent or unclear, and the problem tends to be rather pervasive, which makes it difficult to identify triggers. In such cases, much of the formulation relies on knowledge of the service user's internal world (e.g. their appraisals of the absent activities or behaviours). These CARM formulations can be a good way of clarifying how much is unknown and beginning the process of attempting to collect the knowledge required to better understand the presence or absence of problematic behaviours. Once the formulation has been developed, it is usually clear how care plans can be developed in an attempt to address the problematic behaviour. Typically, it is at the reinforcement or trigger level of the formulation where intervention is most indicated. Positive Behavioural Support plans (PBS; Allen et al., 2005) can also be helpfully integrated here, as CARM is essentially a functional analysis within a social and cognitive context.

EWS-R are another useful output from a CARM formulation, and these can be developed further following the formulation – ideally with the service user as part of a "staying safe" plan. Occasionally, it is noted that behaviour is driven primarily by factors that are not amenable to team intervention (e.g. psychotic phenomena or appraisals in a service user disinclined to engage in therapeutic work). In these cases, the CARM formulation provides information for how to manage risk through external controls.

Assessing and Managing Risks Routinely

We most commonly utilise static-dynamic risk formulations for developing management plans for high-risk problematic behaviours; especially for those behaviours that are historical (e.g. the index offence). These plans should be incorporated into care planning especially when considering changes to leave and moving on (or a reduction in team visits in the community). These are best structured around supporting the service user to manage identified vulnerabilities whilst also supporting and enhancing their strengths. Identified risks can be monitored as part of reassessment and reformulation to reveal changes to the risk profile in response to management and safety planning. As such, we see risk assessment and formulation as an ongoing and cyclical process that is best integrated into a regular programme of assessment, formulation and review.

Summary: Formulations as "Living Documents"

Formulations are not an end in themselves; they exist as part of the process of bringing the team together in the pursuit of developing a better appreciation of the service user's difficulties, needs and strengths. This understanding can be used to inform care planning and design more coherent and effective interventions. As noted at the start of this chapter, formulations should be regarded as a set of hypotheses regarding the factors contributing to the needs of the service user and as such should be held lightly and open to revision in the face of ongoing assessment and updated information. In essence, the formulating process is never complete. Shared formulation functions to provide a good enough map to the challenges and difficulties faced by service users at a given time so as to enable a more effective service response – even if that response is "simply" a better understanding of the person. Formulations need to be adapted to the case-specific and changing needs of the individual service user.

Chapter 4

Risk Assessment in SAFE

Introduction

Understanding and assessing what risks an individual with psychosis may pose to themselves and others is a complex process, not least because (as noted in Chapter 1) psychotic symptoms themselves form only part of the clinical picture. Most focus in the research literature has been on understanding interpersonal violence and suicide. Estimating the likelihood of these risks occurring in the future is at best an inexact science. Estimates for risk behaviour vary depending upon the population studied (e.g. inpatient or community) and the methodology used (see Meaden & Hacker, 2010 for a detailed review). We will never completely know a person's risk for any given behaviour but merely estimate it assuming various conditions and known factors.

Where risk is part of the clinical picture, there is usually a combination of risks including physical (non-sexual) violence/aggression (hitting others, use of weapons); verbal aggression (shouting, insults, threats to harm); suicide (overdose, hanging, jumping, cutting wrists, carbon monoxide poisoning); deliberate self-harm (cutting, stubbing out cigarettes on oneself, ingesting noxious substances); self-neglect/vulnerability from denying oneself personal possessions or food through to exploitation or assault as well as risks to personal safety (e.g. when cooking, crossing the road). Less common are arson and sexual violence (rape, indecent assault, child molestation, exposure, stalking). In this chapter, we will outline how we currently assess for this range of risks and incorporate them into our shared formulations.

Assessment in general can be a powerful way of disentangling clinical problems (see also Meaden & Hacker, 2010; Meaden & Kalidindi, 2015). An over reliance on diagnosis for treatment can be frustrating. Often, in our assessment process as detailed in the following, we identify and agree with the teams we work with, non-mental health-related factors as more important in driving risk behaviours. Good tools orientate clinicians to ask the right questions; though interviews and good quality objective observation are equally important.

DOI: 10.4324/9781003082811-5

A Framework for Assessing Risk

Current methods for assessing risk may be categorised broadly as:

1 Clinical judgement (unstructured judgement based on clinical experience and intuition)
2 SPJ as recommended by the Department of Health (2007) drawing on both clinical experience and the evidence base
3 Actuarial assessment, involving scoring individuals on tools which comprise known risk factors predictive of future risk for particular risk types (e.g. the Violence Risk Appraisal Guide; Quinsey et al., 1998). Actuarial assessment supports adopting an SPJ approach
4 Anamnestic assessment based on what the person has done before and the circumstances involved.

Unstructured clinical judgement rests upon the least empirical support. Whilst some studies have provided support for this approach (e.g. Lidz et al., 1993) the low sensitivity and specificity of these judgements show that clinicians are relatively inaccurate predictors of risk (Skeem & Monahan, 2011). Using risk scales improves accuracy and facilitates clinicians to ask the right questions. Detailed questions regarding a range of factors such as coping skills, engagement in treatment or the ability to form and sustain meaningful relationships form part of the detailed assessment and formulation process. However, it is worth beginning the process with some broad questions to facilitate a shared understanding of the focus for subsequent assessment:

1 *Does the person acknowledge that they can be a risk to themselves or others or that they have engaged in harmful behaviours previously?* If not, then the responsibility will likely fall to others.
2 *Does the person recognise their personal risk factors and the necessity of managing them?* This will be crucial for sustaining more independent living.
3 *Does the person have the skills* (e.g. coping strategies*) to effectively manage their own risk?*
4 *What will they do?* Here we are encouraging all of those involved in the person's care and the individual themselves to think clearly about defining the actual risk behaviours. It is helpful here to ask *what have they done before*, given that the best predictor of future behaviour is past behaviour? Criminal history variables contribute much of the predictive power of actuarial instruments and the predictive accuracy of even the simplest behavioural measures seems to exceed the predictive power of diagnosis (Buchanan, 2008).
5 *Under what circumstances did the behaviour occur?* This often proves difficult to ascertain if the person themselves is not open to discussing it. Notes and records are often vague in this regard. Nevertheless, it is important to

exhaust all known information sources especially if the behaviour (e.g. assault and injury with a weapon) has not occurred for some time with no opportunity to observe the factors potentially driving the behaviour in question directly. Answering this question enables us to understand why the risk behaviour occurs and what factors drive it.

6   *Are the circumstances present now?* Answering this question enables both targeted intervention and management (to reduce the likelihood of harm if the circumstances or factors are present or re-emerge) and promoting positive risk-taking (enabling opportunities for recovery if they are not currently present).

7   *Will the circumstances emerge if the context changes?* (e.g. upon discharge from hospital).

8   *Can the factors driving the behaviour be changed?* This question concerns treatability in terms of how well the person can be engaged in treatment and how effective the treatment is likely to be.

9   *How is the risk best managed?* Here we need to understand (particularly for those who do not respond to treatment or will not engage in it) whether systems can be put in place to monitor and supervise the individual effectively. More intensive community services will likely be needed if for instance the person is discharged from a locked unit. Another consideration here is whether there will be sufficient opportunity to utilise an ESW-R protocol (see Chapter 5) and intervene should signs emerge. Some behaviours may prove highly unpredictable as in the case of behaviours where impulsivity and substance misuse feature. In these cases, it will prove very difficult for intervention to be offered in a sufficiently timely manner.

10   *Are any of the following features present?*

    a   Substance misuse
    b   Personality disorder

Collating information from these questions into a formulation serves several purposes. Firstly, it enables us to construct a narrative or story about how identified factors link together to make each risk behaviour understandable.

Case Illustration: Mark

Mark has an unstable family background characterised by neglect and violence. He views others with suspicion in general as well as having persecutory delusions and command hallucinations. After losing his job as a trainee car mechanic, he became increasingly suspicious of his long-term partner accusing her of having affairs. This led to heated arguments. In order to cope with increased distress, Mark began to use substances again; most notably cocaine. This led to increased feelings of aggression; impulsivity (gambling and other risk-taking behaviours increased) and more frequent command hallucinations. Mark however was noted to be calm though frequently getting up from his chair and checking his phone on a visit from his community team. He denied experiencing any problems. Following a particularly heated argument when his partner threatened to leave Mark, he assaulted her with a kitchen knife. She sustained serious but not life-threatening injuries.

Mark's narrative tells us several things. Firstly, there is a gradual build-up to the assault with several clear factors emerging; namely loss of employment (implicitly involving a loss of status and a valued role) and associated financial impacts, alongside increased relationship problems. Being able to identify **what** the specific factors are provides opportunity to intervene. Objective EWS-R are less easily identified here, but subtle signs of agitation are evident. Finally, a general suspicion of others is a static factor for Mark which is exacerbated by stress and leads to poor coping strategies (e.g. substance use), which in turn increase his impulsivity.

Secondly, formulation enables us to be much clearer about **where** treatment is best targeted; in Mark's case, work around substance use and managing stress and increased psychotic symptoms (multiple attempts to engage him in CBT-P having met with no success). Closer work with Mark's partner is also indicated offering both support and an opportunity (in agreement with Mark) to highlight other EWS-R.

Thirdly, it provides guidance on **when** to intervene; in Mark's case, when he begins to experience stress which exceeds his usual coping strategies (e.g. going to the gym) and when problems in his relationship first occur.

Douglas and Skeem (2005) and Beech and Ward (2004) have usefully identified three types of factors which we have adopted to serve as the basis for our shared risk formulation. Static (including historical) factors cannot, by definition, change over time. They are based on research factors known to predict specific types of risk behaviour (e.g. age, age at first offence, gender, number of previous offences) as well as what the person has done previously. Identifying these helps to answer the question: "How likely is this person, compared to others who have committed an offence, to engage in this behaviour again (within a specified time period)?" However, whilst such static factors tend to be favoured by those wishing to predict risk, clinically derived variables are better placed to offer insights into the mechanisms by which a minority of people with mental disorders act violently (Buchanan, 2008).

Dynamic stable factors are enduring factors linked to the likelihood of risk behaviours occurring. They are termed dynamic as they may change spontaneously or with treatment. Any such change is however likely to be slow; particularly so in this treatment-resistant group. Identifying them involves attempting to understand what factors were involved in previous risk behaviours and how they might be linked to subsequent risk. Such assessment helps to define treatment targets: command hallucinations and substance use, with the aim of reducing risk and promoting positive risk-taking.

Thirdly, dynamic acute factors are more rapidly changing factors. Their presence increases the imminent likelihood of the risk behaviour occurring: increased substance use; isolation; distress; increased preoccupation with delusions; acting on command hallucinations. These factors relate most closely to risk management and when present indicate the need for close supervision and intervention.

It is also important to begin by being very specific and clear regarding the target behaviour for formulation. The static-dynamic framework enables us to draw out the trajectory of a risk behaviour incorporating other risks as relevant. In principle, anything can be a risk factor for a given individual; they are by nature idiosyncratic. Increasingly, we wanted to develop a more structured process in keeping with SPJ principles. The common practice is for one or two individual clinicians to complete structured risk assessments largely in isolation, albeit subsequently sharing the findings with the wider care team. In keeping with our shared principle, we wanted to utilise a tool that involved the whole team as much as possible. We wanted a tool that whilst enabling us to identify relevant factors for risk management and treatment focused also on the individual's strengths, thus promoting a recovery perspective. As highlighted earlier, many risk assessment tools tend to address only specific risk categories such as violence or sexual violence. We wanted a tool that captured the broad range of risks people experiencing psychosis may be vulnerable to. Finally, we wanted to incorporate the process into the team's routine. Reflective practice is the vehicle we chose for this. We chose the START as our tool to address these issues.

The START

The START (Webster et al., 2006) focuses on dynamic factors. It considers the following 20 evidence-based areas in terms of both vulnerabilities (risk) and strengths.

1 Social skills
2 Relationships
3 Occupational
4 Recreational
5 Self-care
6 Mental state
7 Emotional state
8 Substance use
9 Impulse control
10 External triggers
11 Social support
12 Material resources
13 Attitudes

14   Medicine adherence
15   Rule adherence
16   Conduct
17   Insight
18   Plans
19   Coping
20   Treatability

Each area contributes to the formulation of nine risk categories.

1   Violence (verbal and physical aggression)
2   Self-harm
3   Suicide
4   Unauthorised leave
5   Substance abuse
6   Self-neglect
7   Victimisation
8   Sexually inappropriate behaviour
9   Stalking

Three of these are highlighted in terms of acute risk, requiring immediate action if they are judged to be a THREAT (Threats of Harm that are Real, Enactable, Acute and Targeted).

Further judgements are made regarding which areas are vulnerabilities and critical to mediating risks and which areas constitute strengths and may be deemed key items in terms of serving as protective factors which may have a role in reducing risks. Both critical and key items can be care planned (see Chapter 7) with the aim of better managing risks and prompting strengths further. Items are rated in terms of whether they are minimally or not present (0), partially present (1) or definitely present (2) depending on the weighting ascribed to individual evidence-based items comprising each area. The START also includes severity items drawn from a range of tools and supports the use of risk estimates, signature risks with accompanying early signs.

In terms of studies evaluating the utility of the START, several authors have found it to have predictive validity for some risk behaviour outcomes (Braithwaite et al., 2010; Marriott et al., 2017; O'Shea et al., 2014). The majority of studies have focused upon aggression directed towards property and towards others. Methodologies have however been mixed with some researchers collating physical and verbal aggressions into "Any Aggression", with others (Viljoen et al., 2012) combining physical aggression resulting in injury and coercive/violent sexual assaults into "Severe Aggression". The START has been found to have significant predictive validity for verbal aggression (Marriott et al., 2017; O'Shea et al., 2016) and physical aggression (Marriott et al., 2017; O'Shea et al., 2016) up to 12 months, with those designated moderate or high risk presenting an increased likelihood of aggressive behaviours. Strength scores on the START also appear to be associated with risk, with inverted scores being associated will all types of aggression (O'Shea et al., 2016; Marriott et al., 2017), though other studies have failed to find such an association (Braithwaite et al., 2010, Vilijoen et al., 2016). Across these studies, predictive accuracy appears to increase with male gender and decrease with the time over which risk is predicted. Vulnerability scores hold greater predictive validity for all aggression outcomes and appear to possess relative longevity.

In their systematic review of START studies, O'Shea et al. (2014) found good predictive validity for self-harm. However, they found that predictive validity for self-neglect and victimisation was no better than chance. This though should not be surprising since such outcomes represent continuous behaviours and are consequently hard to predict.

Using the START

Reflective Practice Meetings

We meet with as many members of the team as possible once a week for two hours. This typically includes all disciplines; especially those most involved with the persons' care. We aim to complete the START every 6–12 months for each person in a residential unit (depending on type of unit) providing typically 12–18 beds. In community teams, this level of frequency is not possible. Depending upon the type of team, decisions will have to be made regarding which individuals would benefit from a START and shared formulation process. In agreeing who this is most appropriate for, tools such as the CBC-P (Meaden & Hacker, 2010) alongside the RRES (Meaden et al., 2015) can be used as service outcome and profile measures as well as highlighting which individuals pose the greatest risk.

It is helpful when facilitating Reflective Practice meetings to use a projector and to be able to link to the relevant patient information systems used. Prior to the meeting, we endeavour to review the case notes with particular regard to past risk history (for the first START) and collate information regarding incidents for subsequent START (staff collate information using the START incidence record sheet every three months). The Personal, Social, Developmental and Psychiatric History Assessment (Meaden & Hacker, 2010) is a particularly useful tool for collecting and organising relevant information.

To encourage full participation and aid decision-making, we find it helpful to display all of the evidence-based items cited by Webster et al. (2006) in a table format (see Table 4.1). Items can be crossed through if not applicable with remaining items used collectively to rate each area and ascribe a key or critical rating. When repeating the START we have found that the 0–2 rating system gave limited scope for measuring progress or deterioration. We have found it helpful consequently to colour code items.

1   GREEN font colour indicates improvement.

- Strengths being uncrossed and shown in green;
- Vulnerabilities being crossed out and shown in green;
- Green key item indicates a key area that has improved overall.

2   RED font colour indicates a deterioration.

- Strengths being crossed out and shown in red;
- Vulnerabilities being uncrossed out and shown in red;
- Red critical item indicates a critical area that has shown overall deterioration.

3   BLUE font colour indicates sustained improvement.

- Green items from the previous START are turned blue if the improvement has been sustained;
- Green critical and key areas from the previous START are turned blue if the overall improvement in the area has been sustained.

Assessment of risk should not be seen as an end in itself. Any information derived needs to be translated into a formulation showing (in the case of the START) which individual items and areas contribute to a given risk and their stable or dynamic status. The START tool is also intended to be repeated over short periods, through which a dynamic picture of an individual can be developed (Webster et al., 2006). This also supports our need-adapted treatment principle (Meaden & Hacker, 2010) allowing changing needs to be considered.

Incorporating SAFE Shared Formulations

Generating shared formulations using the START as noted in Chapter 2 is embedded within our team reflective practice sessions. The original version of the START includes options for recording signature risk signs, making specific risk estimates, noting current management measures and providing a risk formulation alongside any health concerns/medical issues and test results. These elements of the START seemed natural to us as both fitting with the SAFE approach and affording the opportunity for making SAFE adaptations. Most notably, the signature risk signs fitted well with our EWS-R methodology whilst the formulation section fitted well with our emphasis on formulation. For management plans we felt it important to focus on the potential for recovery and have consequently adopted Positive Behaviour Plans (see Chapter 7). We have steered away from making risk estimates since as discussed earlier even the best estimates are little

Table 4.1 Evidence-Based START Strength and Vulnerability Items for Each Area

START areas	Strengths	Vulnerabilities
1 Social Skills	· Pleasant · Polite · Joins in group activities · Initiates conversations · Good communication skills · Socially appropriate behaviour · Feels satisfaction in social situations	· Avoids social situations · Isolated/Withdrawn/Shy · Loner · Difficult to engage · Lacks manners · Does not communicate well · Immature · Intrusive
2 Relationships	· Empathetic · Considerate · Reciprocal relating · Values and builds friendships and close relationships · Gets along with others · Is able to feel close to others · Is satisfied with interpersonal relationships · Gauges how actions affect others · Forms close relationships and forms therapeutic alliances	· Superficial · Unreliable · Aloof · Inconsiderate · Takes advantage of others · Manipulates · Provokes · Objectifies others · Derives little satisfaction from interpersonal relationships · Deceptive · Unfriendly · Unable to sustain relationships · Lacks empathy · Does not form therapeutic alliances · Is taken advantage of in abusive relationships
3 Occupational	· Understands the value of education and work · Seeks out opportunities · Is willing to be advised · Consents to starting out at a level appropriate to existing experience and skills · Reliable · Does assignments on time · Has good work habits · Show initiative in the classroom/on the job	· Has no apparent interest in education or work · Fails to follow through when opportunities are presented · Does not show up · Consistently late or does not attend at all · Requires inordinate amounts of help to complete the most minimal of tasks · Refuses participation

4 Recreational	· Aware of recreational opportunities · Uses leisure time constructively · Enjoys recreational activities · Plans activities for self and others · Willing to be helped to develop interests and hobbies · Takes regular physical exercise	· Largely sedentary · Does not want to engage in recreational pursuits · Refuses to participate in new activities and pro-social projects · Has few if any hobbies or interests · Does not undertake regular physical exercise
5 Self-care	· Carries out basic personal hygiene · Maintains personal space in satisfactory condition · Appropriately dressed · Normal sleep patterns · Normal eating patterns · Accepts health teaching	· Personal hygiene is maintained at less than minimal levels only · Personal space is disordered and unclean · Dresses in idiosyncratic or inappropriate fashion · Does not follow health teaching · Abnormal sleep patterns · Abnormal eating patterns · Abnormal fluid intake
6 Mental state	· Maintains stability, focus and flexibility in thought · Demonstrates coherent, logical, abstract and innovative thought	· Disorganised thinking · Obsessional or perseverative thoughts · Delusions · Hallucinations · Poverty of ideation · Flight of idea · Confusion, disorientation · Impaired attention and memory functions
7 Emotional state	· Good spirits · Sense of humour · Hopeful · Emotionally resilient · Ability to experience emotions · Mood appropriate to circumstances	· Depressed · Inappropriately elevated mood · Labile · Pessimistic · Emotionally withdrawn · Lethargic · Feelings of worthlessness · Hopelessness · Irritable · Angry · Emotionally restricted

Table 4.1 (Continued)

START areas	Strengths	Vulnerabilities
8 Substance use	· Abstains · Drinks in moderation · Restricts intake · Remains responsible · Respects pertinent laws · Protect others from ill effects (i.e. is aware of the consequences of irresponsible use) · Accepting of treatment (if needed)	· Adverse effects on self or others when under influence · Uses illegal substances · Indiscriminate intake · Takes prescription/non-prescription drugs improperly · Denies need for treatment (if indicated) · Use is out of control · Intoxicated · Dependent
9 Impulse control	· Restrained · Calm · Contained · Deliberate · Controlled · Thinks before acting · Considers consequences · Tolerates frustration	· Overwrought · Erratic · Out-of-control · Excited · Risk-taking · Impulsive · Acts on spur of moment · Does not anticipate consequences · Poor frustration tolerance
10 External triggers	· Pro-social associates · Suitable living conditions · Acts independently of changing circumstances and pressures · Is not easily influenced to act irresponsibly or unlawfully	· Influenced by disruptive peers · Susceptible to unsuitable environments · Affected by specific destabilisers and changing demands in the environment · Access to weapons
11 Social support	· Social support from family, friends, professionals and other adequate social network	· Non-availability or non-acceptance of social support · Inadequate social network

12 Material resources	· Adequate means/income · No financial drains · Responsible management of finances · Stable and satisfactory housing	· Financially restricted · Irresponsible management of finances · Large debts · Resists being helped with financial planning · Poor or unstable housing · Does not have money for food, transportation, healthcare and affordable diversions and entertainments
13 Attitudes	· Pro-community · Appropriately self-confident · Respectful · Forgiving · Remorseful (if appropriate) · Honest · Forthright · Shows concern for others · Tolerant of others · Respects legitimate authority · Appropriate self-esteem · Accepting	· Pro-criminal · Grandiose · Callous · Remorseless · Narcissistic · Selfish · Collusive · Hostile · Dishonest · Lacks empathy · Aggressive attributional style · Entitled · Takes offence easily · Resentful · Self-esteem difficulties
14 Medication adherence	· Responsible medication management · Makes effort to understand the function of prescribed medications and how side effects can be minimised or eliminated	· Does not take prescribed medication or will accept only particular kinds · Does not follow recommended regimen
15 Rule adherence	· Obeys rules and legally stipulated conditions · Makes effort to see the point of restrictions · Provides bodily samples as requested	· Does not attempt to understand the points behind the rules and conditions · Disobeys rules · Grudgingly complies with conditions · Refuses to cooperate with urine, blood and other routine tests · Substitutes samples

(Continued)

Table 4.1 (Continued)

START areas	Strengths	Vulnerabilities
16 Conduct	· Accepts responsibility · Obeys laws · Respects property · Punctual · Creates a positive atmosphere · Is considerate · Is attentive to safety, comfort and care of self or others · Adjusts behaviour according to social context	· Escapes · Barricades · Threatens · Starts fires · Destroys property · Assaults · Steals · Disrupts · Sets others up for failure · Complains repeatedly about staff without justification · Insults · Teases · Is obnoxious · Sexual conduct is unacceptable · Intimidates · Bullies · Makes racist, sexist or other such comments · Interferes with co-clients' assessments, treatments and management · Engages in harm to self
17 Insight	· Aware of strengths and limitations · Makes connections between thought and action · Applies facts to own state and circumstances · Acknowledges mental, personality or substance use disorder and (if present) the need for interventions · Understands personal risk factors and necessity of managing them · Recognises signs of relapse at an early stage	· Not self-aware · Fails to appreciate motivation behind own actions · Denies mental, personality or substance use disorder and (if present) the need for interventions · Does not identify and/or manage personal risk factors · No recognition of early signs of relapse

18 Plans	· Socially acceptable · Realistic · Focused · Future-oriented · Goal-directed · Has plans to achieve short- and long-term goals	· Goals are absent or vague · Unrealistic · Unacceptable · Has neither short-term plans nor long-term goals
19 Coping	· Solves problems effectively and independently · Seeks help and uses it · Finds positive aspects in otherwise upsetting or worrying circumstances · Manages stress · Resilient · Adaptable · Manages transitions satisfactorily	· Unable to solve problems without considerable assistance · Disintegrates under pressure · Unable to marshal personal resources at the time of crises · Becomes immobilised or defeated under challenge · Lacks resiliency · Difficulty adapting · Finds it hard to deal with crises, transitions and real, imagined or anticipated losses
20 Treatability	· Participates in programmes and treatment likely to be of benefit · Cooperative · Wants to succeed · Not satisfied merely to "look good" or to be viewed as a "model client" · Responds well to biological, social and psychological treatments	· Perceives no point in attempting change · Unengaged · Uncooperative · When more or less obliged to participate in programmes, merely "goes through the motions" · Unresponsive to biological, social and psychological treatments

Adapted and reproduced with kind permission from St Jospeh's Healthcare: Webster, C. D., Martin, M., Brink, J., Nicholls, T. L., & Middleton, C. (2004). *Short-Term assessment of risk and treatability (START)*. St. Josephs Healthcare, Hamilton and British Columbia Mental Health and Addiction Services.

better than chance. Our focus remains on formulation to guide positive risk-taking decisions.

Static-dynamic formulations are particularly helpful when formulating longer-term historical risks. They also help the team to understand how factors link together to result in a given risk behaviour. However, we found that team members struggled to separate out and identify appropriate treatment targets from these narratives. In an effort to clarify the key potential intervention and management targets for current risks and problem behaviours, we integrated our CARM formulation (see Appendices 2 and 3) in a narrative format. Combining these two shared formulations alongside the START tool rating has enabled us to considerably reduce the time it would take to complete each of these formulations as separate processes as well as collating them all in one place.

Case Illustration: Sara

Definition of the Risk Behaviour

Punching staff and other residents in the face and kicking them on the shins

Static-Dynamic Shared Formulation

Sara had a neglectful and abusive childhood. She was bullied at school and truanted much of the time. She began hearing voices at an early age and these special spirits became her friends and "life guides". Sara can be seen to become increasingly verbally hostile during the day if things do not go her way (being refused requests and being picked on by other service users). Subsequently, Sara can become physically aggressive towards staff and others when she feels she is being treated unfairly or when her requests are persistently denied.

Shared CARM Formulation

Vulnerability Factors:

- Paranoia – jumps to conclusions (cognitive bias) – feeling targeted and persecuted against;
- Voices (benevolent voices advising that others are talking down to her);
- Poor frustration tolerance;
- Perceives others as not caring – sensitive to abandonment and rejection;
- Low self-esteem;
- Racist attitudes.

Setting Events (Internal and External):

- Black and ethnic minority staff on shift;[1]
- Trading with peers and being "ripped off" by them;
- Being prompted by staff to get up and carry out self-care;
- Preoccupation with voices.

Triggers (Internal and External):

- When requests/perceived needs are denied (especially by BME staff);
- When peers laugh at her for complaining about earlier trades;
- When Sara feels she is being neglected.

Reinforcers (Internal and External):

- BME staff avoid her;
- Voices say "that will teach them" and "don't take anymore shit";
- Peers give her extra items (e.g. cans of coke).

Protective Factors:

- Good relationship with some staff;
- Recognises behaviours work against goals of achieving more independent living (identified from Recovery Goal Planning Interview, Meaden & Hacker, 2010).

Some risks are however much harder to formulate using these methods. Most notably, self-neglect which we describe as a continuous behaviour or set of behaviours. Here, we may be able to identify only some factors of the formulation.

Definition of the Risk Behaviour:

Unkempt/dishevelled appearance; dirty clothes/refusing to change clothing, dirty/untidy bedroom; offensive odour.

Static-Dynamic Shared Formulation:

Sara has a long-standing history of self-neglect. She ignores prompts from staff stating "fuck off and leave me alone". Sara had few possessions or new clothes growing up and lived in a squat for a long time. She spends a lot of time responding to her voices and has little interest in leaving the unit to go out into the community. She responds poorly when staff approach her.

Shared CARM Formulation

Vulnerability Factors:

- Early deprivation and neglect;
- Homelessness;
- Few friends and a loner – possibly less concerned about the opinions of others.

Setting Events (Internal and External):

None evident

Triggers (Internal and External):

None evident

Reinforcers (Internal and External):

- Able to spend more time interacting with her voices;
- Some staff may take her insults personally and this may change their interaction with her;
- Sara often picks up on this, leading to a further deterioration in her interactions with staff.

Protective Factors:

- Despite personal history, Sara has built a good relationship with some staff;
- Recognises behaviours that work against goals of achieving more independent living.

In Sara's case our shared static-dynamic formulation appears more helpful in understanding this behaviour. It is understandable and requires a care plan focused on engagement with and developing the ability to sustain caring relationships. The aim here is to enable Sara to accept care and learn, thereby to care about herself. The TBCT plan here is aimed at promoting staff compassion and understanding to enable non-judgemental interactions. At the same time, Sara will need to be communicated about non-acceptance of any racist attitudes and abuse.

Agreeing Treatment Targets

The START itself along with our formulation processes inevitably generates a great many potential care plans (see Chapter 10). Also, we draw together outcomes from the Recovery Goal Planning Interview or RGPI (Meaden & Hacker, 2010), as well as our SLF, which highlights the key barriers to recovery (see Chapter 3). Risk assessment and shared formulation findings most relevant to identifying intervention targets are the following.

1   Key items
2   Critical items
3   Setting events (via EWS-R)
4   Triggers
5   Reinforcers

In determining how best to utilise all of this information, it is helpful to firstly ask whether the service user can be engaged in individual one-to-one treatment. Here, we have found two items from the start particularly helpful. Firstly, "Insight", which covers the extent to which the individual can recognise and understand the necessity for managing early signs of relapse and risk. Secondly, "Treatability", which concerns the person's ability to engage with and benefit from social, biological and psychological interventions. The RRES is also helpful here: does the person only score in the domain of agreeing with treatment and basic relationships or do they show evidence of more active participation? A lack of strengths in these areas will likely mean that team efforts will have to focus instead on intervening when, for instance, early signs are present, as well as adapting the social environment, to better manage setting events. Interventions will also be needed at the reinforcer level utilising behavioural interventions based on differential reinforcement principles.

In agreeing with what to target, it is helpful to focus on a smaller number of areas and to avoid overlapping and competing efforts (a need-adapted treatment principle, see Meaden & Hacker, 2010). Consideration should be given to how severe and acute current risks are. THREAT-rated items on the START should be prioritised. Some areas will be harder to change, such as antisocial attitudes compared to engagement with recreational activities. It is good both for the motivation of the team and the individual to incorporate recreational items (especially those where strengths are also evident) into the care planning process.

Summary

We have not attempted here to provide a detailed account of risk assessment in psychosis. Indeed, there are many excellent texts covering risk assessment in general in more detail. What we have offered here is our revised approach to risk assessment in SAFE. It is an integrated process incorporating team assessment, formulation and goal setting into a shared process. In Chapter 12, we look at how

START is used to capture meaningful change and better enable services to target their efforts more accurately.

Note

1 We subsequently devise ESW-R plans to address these setting events.

Chapter 5

Using Early Warning Signs in SAFE

Introduction

Identifying Early Warning Signs of Psychotic relapse (EWS-P) is now well established in clinical practice. Whilst various methodologies exist, the common purpose is to be able to spot when early signs first emerge and engage in actions designed to prevent a relapse. When working with those with complex mental health and behavioural needs it is necessary to adopt a broad definition of the term relapse as many of those we work with have persistent and enduring symptoms. Our working description therefore encompasses both an exacerbation of psychotic symptoms and a decrease in functioning which may also require hospitalisation (Gaebel & Riesbeck, 2007; Vigod et al., 2015).

Despite advances in biopsychosocial treatment, relapse in people with a diagnosis of schizophrenia remains common, and this risk cannot be eliminated (Emsley et al., 2013; Linszen et al., 1998). As many as 80% of people diagnosed with a first episode of psychosis will experience a recurrence of symptoms with the potential for a second relapse as high as 78% (Emsley et al., 2012; Robinson et al., 1999; Watt et al., 1983; Wiersma et al., 1998). In those who have received a diagnosis of psychosis lasting for many years and show low remission in their symptoms for a prolonged period, multiple relapses are common over the course of their mental health journey (Emsley et al., 2013). Vigod et al. (2013) highlight the value of early intervention for relapse prevention, particularly given that successive relapses have been linked to cognitive decline and reductions in social functioning (Wiersma et al., 1998) alongside the economic costs associated with relapse (Schizophrenia Commission, 2016). Whilst our primary objective in SAFE is to reduce risk behaviour and thereby reduce barriers to recovery, any increase or return of psychotic symptoms may well be implicated in risk. EWS-P research and practice also brings with it a useful set of principles which we have adopted for our EWS-R methodology (Meaden et al., 2013).

Relapse Prevention

Docherty et al. (1978) have argued that psychotic relapses occur in a predictive order, indicating that each service user has their own unique relapse experience.

DOI: 10.4324/9781003082811-6

This pattern or signature of symptoms and experiences has been termed a "relapse signature" (Birchwood et al., 2000). Mapping and monitoring of the emergence and course of this signature supports the targeting of interventions designed to prevent or delay relapse. Methods designed to achieve this build on the notion of the stress-vulnerability model in psychosis (Zubin & Spring, 1977) and typically involve the identification of idiosyncratic stress triggers and signs which can be further categorised into early, middle and late stages and a set of coping strategies developed linked to each stage. Gillespie (2015) has provided a useful framework for using EWS-P approaches with hard-to-reach-and-treat populations.

EWS-P With Hard-to-Reach Populations

Research has suggested that relapse prevention can help with delaying a relapse, increase functioning over time, increase medication compliance and help service users gain a better understanding of their psychosis and how to manage it (Lobban et al., 2010; Lee et al., 2010; Pontin et al., 2009; Peters et al., 2011). However, Gillespie (2015) found no published studies looking at the effectiveness of relapse prevention specifically with hard-to-engage populations, and to our knowledge this remains the case. Indeed, it is known that implementing psychosocial interventions (e.g. CBT-P) within this population group has been difficult due to several factors including lack of dedicated time, lack of supervision, the difficulty of implementing the structured nature of the interventions and the predominance of the medical model (Williams, 2008; Griffiths & Harrias, 2008). In service users who are hard to reach, their level of engagement in relapse prevention work may prove challenging for a number of reasons. They may not agree that they have a mental illness, may be in a crisis or in the middle of a relapse. When stable, they may struggle to recall previous episodes of relapse, whilst others may always be experiencing a persistent level of distressing psychotic experiences (see Gillespie, 2015). As such, we can refine and adapt the relapse prevention process for people who are hard to reach by harnessing the system around the person through team-based interventions and group-based work.

Team-Based Relapse Prevention Planning

Working with the wider MDT is the cornerstone of SAFE and may be extended to include family networks. Teams and families have useful information and insights into the stress triggers, presentation patterns and potential coping strategies that may be useful in ameliorating relapse. Collating information from these sources will enhance the validity of any relapse plan, increasing the likelihood that they will work across as many situations and contexts as possible. In our experience, initial psychoeducation for all of those involved in developing the plan around the key principles of relapse is usually necessary. The "stress-vulnerability" model of Zubin and Spring (1977) offers a non-stigmatising and straightforward way of conceptualising relapse. Within this model, biopsychosocial stress is hypothesised to act as a trigger to onset of psychosis (e.g. drug use, money worries, family problems). The term psychosis may be usefully relabelled to match with the service users' view of their journey, for example how they arrived in hospital. Even disengaged service users are usually motivated to avoid further admissions. In keeping with our focus on engagement we have renamed the EWS-P plan as Stress Management Plan. Here the emphasis is on enabling the service user to manage their stress. It helpfully moves away from the notion of relapse and by implication "illness" models and begins a shared dialogue. In Rakeem's case discussed later, we move beyond whether his reactions are the result of a psychotic illness and to a position of helping him avoid relapse and conflict with others. A shared dialogue does however not involve condoning the use of violence where this is part of the relapse process. We avoid being drawn into the rights and wrongs of such actions and instead focus on their consequences. In Rakeem's case, these will likely continue if nothing changes.

Objective and external observable stress triggers that build the potential to relapse can be simple to identify; however, when not involving the service user, it is more effective to focus on observable signs of relapse (e.g. talking to oneself as a sign of auditory hallucinations; raising one's voice and shouting as signs of anger) rather than speculating on potential internal (and unobservable) signs. If not directly involving the service user, then the monitoring of early signs and the delivery of effective support or coping strategies need to be carefully considered and planned. However, it is our experience that even the most disengaged service users will agree to view and offer their opinion on plans even if they do not agree to be involved in their development.

Case Illustration: Rakeem

Rakeem is in his mid-forties, has a diagnosis of schizoaffective disorder and is currently on the caseload of an AOT. He lives with his mother and has a history of multiple hospital admissions, often associated with worsening persecutory paranoia and verbal aggression towards his mother. More recently, he was admitted following a physical fight in a supermarket carpark where he accused another shopper of staring at him. Rakeem has denied that he has a problem, arguing that the problem is other people seeking to "start trouble". He has explained that there is "no point" in relapse prevention work as there is nothing he can do to prevent others from "starting trouble" and being taken into hospital as a result.

Rakeem's care coordinator and the team psychologist explained to Rakeem that they would be meeting his mother to develop a stress management plan to help him to remain out of hospital, which he agreed to but declined to engage with. Over several meetings in the family home with Rakeem's mother, and a review of the case notes, a relapse pattern was developed. This focussed on Rakeem's enduring concerns that people have malicious intent towards him, often exacerbated by world events and general life stressors (such as meeting new people).

A management plan that involved Rakeem's mother and team, with clearly observable signs and symptoms, was developed over several meetings (see Table 5.1). A prototype set of coping strategies was developed, split between those that would be best delivered by the team and those delivered by his mother. Rakeem reviewed the plan and suggested some new strategies and advised on wording he would find less troublesome should he be becoming more anxious, suspicious or paranoid. Rakeem reported that he was satisfied for other people to try these but was steadfast in his belief that these would not work. He agreed to take a copy of the coping strategies so that he could remind himself of the plan, which he put on the inside of his wardrobe door.

Enhancing Engagement Through a Group Format for Relapse Prevention

Whilst traditionally relapse prevention for psychosis is completed on an individual basis with the service user, family or team, Gillespie (2015) identified the benefits of a group-based approach. We subsequently developed a manualised group to help deliver the psychoeducation components of relapse prevention planning within particularly hard-to-reach groups (Fox & Sharp, 2018). This approach utilises the shared experiences of the group and the notion of stress vulnerability (Zubin & Spring, 1977) to destigmatise the process and therefore enhance engagement. This is particularly important given the recognition of the role of shame (and associated avoidance) that is often experienced alongside psychosis (Carden et al., 2018).

Our manualised group programme comprises seven sessions:

1 Introduction and consideration of what I'm like when I'm well (me at my best)
2 What is the stress vulnerability bucket?
3 What does my stress vulnerability bucket look like?
4 The effects of stress: early warning signs planning
5 Coping strategies
6 Individual sessions: complete relapse preventions plan
7 Ending: putting it all together and group endings.

We strongly recommend that all sessions are run by the same staff members to promote the development of trusting therapeutic relationships and enhance engagement. The notion of a psychosis continuum (Van Os et al., 2000) underpins the group philosophy, while language that is non-pathologising is encouraged (e.g. "experiences" rather than "symptoms"). Similarly, facilitators share (in a safe and boundaried manner) their own experiences of stress in an effort to normalise experiences, reduce shame and stigma and encourage sharing of information relevant to relapse prevention planning.

The group uses a variety of activities, worksheets and games alongside frequent breaks to enhance engagement and work across sensory modalities, which also accommodates for difficulties in concentration and motivation, such as those

Table 5.1 Rakeem's Team-Based Stress Management Plan

Possible Stress Triggers		
Drinking alcohol during the day	Problems with benefits	Changes in medication
Changing care coordinator	Meeting new people (e.g. training, work)	News events about terrorists

Early Signs and Ways of Managing my Stress	
What will people see?	What can people do to help?
Early: • Staying up late at night (past 1a.m.) • Talking less to mum • Spending lots more time in my room • Not going out so much • Not eating so regularly or ordering more takeaways	**Mum:** • Ask me how I am feeling (but do not keep going on if I don't look like I want to talk) • Offer to make me my favourite tea and catch up with me over this • Use the "problem solving" techniques to help me work through any daily hassles • Let the team know if I am worried about any problems I am having (e.g. benefits) but tell me when you're doing this **Team:** • Offer to take me out for a coffee or tea to Coffee Lounge • Check in with me and mum on the phone to see if there is any support we need
Middle: • Short and sharp in discussions • Watching more factual ("conspiracy") shows on TV/the internet • Talking more about people outside of the family • Pacing more in my room • Spending time looking out of the window (checking outside of the house)	**Mum:** • Let the team know any concerns I have **Team:** • Weekly check in with my mum to make sure she feels supported • Remind mum about the carer support services • Daily contact with me on the phone to check my concerns/reassure me about my worries
Late: • Reversed sleeping pattern (asleep during day, up at night) • Raising my voice more in conversations • Looking tired, pacing and agitated • Frequently annoyed on return home from trips out	**Mum:** • Try to keep daily routine • Offer me a cup of tea in the morning Team: • Discuss respite break with me (1–2 weeks) • Come over for daily medication checks but remind me why you're coming (send a text before so I know you're coming) • Discuss inpatient admission

associated with cognitive deficits. Work is ongoing to monitor the outcomes of this group format, but initial pilot work suggests that this can be a potentially useful method for establishing the notion of relapse prevention plans and enhancing engagement in the process of their development (Fox & Sharp, 2018).

Early Warning Signs of Risk

EWS-R are relevant in understanding and trying to predict risk and more generally in relation to understanding the function of challenging and risk behaviours. Moreover, they are helpful in further structuring clinical judgement drawing on relevant known factors as appropriate. Predicting risk (as noted in Chapter 3) presents a continuous challenge and is important when deciding whether to reduce or remove a service user's restrictions such as whether someone is ready to be discharged from hospital or have their leave increased. Clinical judgement alone has its limitations and is prone to missing crucial information, as it is influenced by feelings towards the person and to normal and subconscious biases that all clinicians may have (Kahneman & Tversky, 1979).

Using the principles from EWS-P, Meaden and Hacker (2010) observed that hard-to-reach service users also seem to have a unique pattern of relapse when it comes to monitoring their risk behaviours. Meaden et al. (2013) tested this methodology as applied to risk and found relevant early warning signs of risk could be reliably identified and monitored by multidisciplinary staff. They moreover found that in order to be clinically useful, the signs and target behaviour required clear operational definitions and would need to be reliably monitored. Their findings highlighted how the approach showed potential for the targeting of interventions to prevent future aggression in inpatient settings. The results further supported the notion that EWS-R method used has the potential for identifying acute risk and hence prevention of actual aggression.

EWS-R for Active and Passive Behaviours

Our approach to categorising behaviours as broadly either active or passive enables us to decide which are best formulated using EWS-R. Active behaviours are more relevant for EWS-R since they are more likely to have observable signs (to both the individual and the staff). By contrast, passive behaviours tend to be continuous, making it difficult to devise an early warning signs plan as the behaviour may be continuously present in the absence of identifiable triggers. EWS-R are a crucial part of both our CARM formulation (for active behaviours) and our shared static-dynamic risk formulation. The EWS-R themselves constitute a mini formulation or further level of formulation and may be used as a stand-alone piece of work.

Case Illustration: Sarah

Sarah has heard voices since she was a teenager. These voices make both positive and negative comments about her. When things are going wrong in Sarah's life, her critical voice would become prominent and tell Sarah that she is useless, no good to anyone and that it would be better if she was not here. The voices would sometimes tell Sarah to cut herself and Sarah would respond by superficially cutting her wrist in partial compliance of these commands. On another occasion, following an argument with her boyfriend, Sarah would cut her arms as a way of managing her emotional distress. Sarah would also cut herself if she was having a difficult period in her life and the voices were repeatedly telling her that she was "no good" and "a failure".

On the surface, all three of Sarah's self-harm behaviours look the same; however, they all have different functions. The former and latter of the examples have psychotic features while the second example is driven by emotional distress. Two of these behaviours are voice related but serve different functions: one to comply with voice commands and one as a means of managing emotional distress from persistent derogatory voice comments.

EWS-R crucially underpins our TBCT approach. These are not readily elicited during team formulation sessions and usually require a separate piece of work ideally combined with a TBCT care plan. EWS-R consist of the external observable signs of both internal and external setting events. These often-subtle changes in a person can escalate slowly or quickly into a risk behaviour. Unlike EWS-P, the subtle signs do not always present as dysphoric in nature, but like ESW-P they are often idiosyncratic.

Developing an EWS-R Plan

Ideally, this work should be carried out with the service user and their family. However, with hard-to-reach populations this is often not possible. In these cases, we default to devising EWS-P plans with the MDT. Sometimes, relevant information can be elicited during reflective practice sessions. These sessions moreover help highlight risk and challenging behaviours that require EWS-R planning; however, it is often necessary to obtain further information. Members of the MDT most closely involved with the service user can usefully examine historical information from clinical notes and may come together to complete the EWS-R checklist (Meaden & Hacker, 2010). This usefully categorises signs into three types.

Contextual Signs: these are factors that may function as external setting events, such as arguments with family; boredom; lack of activities; changes in staff or other service users. They can set the scene for challenging or risk behaviours to occur.

Visual Signs: these are aspects of internal setting events that can be objectively observed by others (e.g. increased voice activity might be observed by the person withdrawing to their room and playing the radio noisily).

Verbal Signs: these are aspects of internal setting events that can be observed only through verbal interactions between the service user and others. For example increases in hostility and suspicion might be observed by negative comments about a particular staff member being made; paranoia about other service users may manifest as shouting or making insults directed towards them.

The checklist items are not exclusive but serve as a starting point. Care should be taken to refine checklist-endorsed items and individualise them. EWS-R and EWS-P may be very similar for some individuals as they relate to understanding a given risk behaviour. Teams can also use the Challenging Behaviour Record Sheet for Psychosis or CBRS-P (Meaden & Hacker, 2010) to identify distal triggers.

As with EWS-P, signs can be usefully categorised into early, middle and late. The team should also document what the service user is like when they are well or stable (typical presentation). This will help staff and their families to identify changes in behaviour that are atypical and potentially indicate the imminence of the risk behaviour.

Appropriate strategies to be employed in the presence of each early sign stage (early, middle and late) should be agreed next. Ideally, this is best done in conjunction with the service user as part of the process of recovery: being able to identify and manage their own risk factors. This part of the process can also help identify if the service user has appropriate coping strategies and when best to use them to prevent risk or challenging behaviours from occurring. If they do not have many effective coping strategies, work will need to be undertaken to enable them to develop these. These can in turn form part of a TBCT care plan with the staff team prompting and supporting the service user to utilise coping strategies when appropriate (i.e. in the presence of early signs).

Post-incident, EWS-R should be reviewed with the service user, staff who witnessed the incident and family members (if relevant) to establish if they were accurate indicators. Any changes can then be made to fine-tune the process.

Case Study: Steve

Steve has a history of smoking cannabis but has always denied doing so and has stated that he even declined it when it was offered to him on the unit. Steve denies having a mental illness and struggles to see or acknowledge any deterioration or improvements in his mental state. When Steve smokes cannabis, his paranoia increases, he believes that his family are out to steal from him and harm him, and he has been known to physically attack them and throw furniture around the house. During one such incident the family called the police. Police officers attending the incident were assaulted as Steve believed that the police were also out to harm him. His index offence involved punching a police officer in a fight (he was intoxicated at the time) for which he was arrested and sent to prison. Shortly afterwards he was sent to a medium secure forensic mental health unit. When he was stabilised, he was transferred to a locked rehabilitation unit.

Many of the incidents of violence can be attributed to poor control of his symptoms, but some are related to his personality and attitude towards authority.

Due to Steve's ongoing low-level of paranoia, Steve's behaviour towards his peers and staff members can at times be viewed as challenging. He is verbally aggressive and scowls at some of his peers. He has also been observed imitating staff members, laughing and mocking them. Steve will steal his peer's food and cigarettes and later be seen selling these back to them. Steve also makes some unwanted physical contact with his peers in the form of flicking their ears, tapping them on their heads and pretending to punch them and shouting loudly to peers who are more introverted and timid.

When out on escorted leave, Steve would request to make unscheduled visits to other locations. When this is declined, Steve was known to abscond or walk off and staff would have to follow him, which later results in his leave being suspended. When staff talked to Steve about these behaviours, he initially blames others, or states that he is doing this because others were provoking him. Steve can also minimise his behaviours by saying that he is only joking or that he was just messing about. Steve would say not all staff members see his behaviour as a problem and he would be confused as to why some staff members allowed him to visit other venues whilst some did not. With additional support, Steve has some reflective capacity to understand how his behaviour is sometimes seen as unhelpful. However, he claims also that he cannot help his behaviour (indicating his behaviour is impulsive). Steve moreover believes that some members of staff are "out to get" him and are always looking for ways to get him into trouble.

Narrative CARM formulations were completed for Steve as part of the START process. These were subsequently used to inform which behaviours might benefit from further EWS-R work. The most frequent and, from the staff's perspective, most difficult of these behaviours involved physical aggression towards others. These also acted as a significant barrier for Steve getting leave.

Following a subsequent reflective practice discussion that focused on reviewing his CARM formulation, it was agreed that the psychologist would attempt to work both individually with Steve and with the team to try and address these behaviours. Steve was initially unsure about being involved with psychology, but he said he wanted to be seen as cooperative and keep his leave, so he agreed to engage in this piece of work.

Stage 1: Agreeing and Clarifying the Target Behaviour

The team felt that Steve would benefit from some support around managing his active behaviour broadly defined as physical aggression towards others. These episodes generally, yet not always, followed Steve being declined certain things like extra food or leave. Clearly, therefore other factors were involved. It was evident from completing the START process, CARM and narrative static-dynamic formulations that Steve could begin by being verbally aggressive towards others before escalating into physical violence. The team agreed that the operationally defined behaviour they would like to complete in an EWS-R was:

"Steve being violent towards others – punching or hitting them"

Steve's Narrative CARM Formulation

Vulnerability Factors:

Diagnosis of paranoid schizophrenia (which he does not agree with);
Paranoid delusions – believes past gang members are after him and that staff are being paid by them to harm him;
Ideas of reference from the TV (sending signals and messages – we are watching you, we know where you are, we will catch up with you soon);
General paranoid beliefs: staff laughing at him;
Domestic abuse in the family;
Grown up with pro-criminal associates;
History of violence: convicted for committing grievous bodily harm;
Antisocial personality traits;
Difficulties managing emotions;
Substance abuse history;
Poor frustration tolerance;
Impulsive;
Low self-esteem;
Low agency of control;
Using food to self soothe;
Diabetes.

External Setting Events:

Being refused midnight snacks;
Watching TV news about gangs and drugs;
Being around a peer who targets him;

Going to the city centre with new and inexperienced staff;
Going to the shops on unescorted leave;
Receiving benefits.

Internal Setting Events:

Increased feelings of paranoia;
Poor sleep;
Hypervigilance – looking out for signs that peer and staff want to hurt him.

External Triggers:

Requests being denied (e.g. home leave, food, cigarettes, going to shops);
Staff approach – not realising when to disengage, tone of voice, making him
feel undermined;
Remote control being taken off him;
Peers mocking him or not listening to him.

Internal Triggers:

Feeling vulnerable and the need to protect himself;
Believes members of staff are targeting him;
Feeling provoked;
Feeling undermined and not listened to;
Feeling a rush of anger.

External Reinforcers:

Staff and peers leave him alone;
Not being challenged about his behaviour.

Internal Reinforcers:

Prevents perceived abuse from others;
Feelings of power, dominance and control;
Release of emotions;
Wanting to make people feel the way he is feeling.

The clinical notes were further reviewed to examine previous incidents of when
Steve had punched or hit others. His named nurse completed the EWS-R checklist for this behaviour to help identify external observable signs of both the likely
internal and external setting events (the distant triggers).

Stage 2: Identifying Triggers, Setting Events and Reinforcers

The assistant psychologist identified all recorded past incidents from the case notes in relation to this specific risk behaviour and all possible immediate triggers and setting events that could have contributed to it as well as identifying the staff's responses and Steve's explanation (post incident). Information was also collated from the CBRS-P.

The named nurse and two healthcare assistants used information from the EWS-R checklist to identify contextual, verbal and visual signs that Steve may exhibit when he demonstrated this behaviour. All members of the team involved thus far then met together to collate the information in the EWS-R plan to take it back to the team and service user/family member to discuss further.

Stage 3: Sharing the EWS-R Formulation

In order to prevent the behaviour from occurring, it was vital that all staff and ideally the service user understood and recognised the presence of these early signs and changed their behaviour accordingly. Examples included practising relaxation and spending less time alone in his room.

Steve's named nurse met with him to go through the EWS-R. Steve said that he would become angry and hit out at people when he was denied food or when people said "no" to him. He felt that it was the staff's role to take care of him and listen to his requests as this is *"what they are paid to do!"*. When he felt dismissed or undermined, Steve would lash out. He also felt he was being targeted by another peer and felt his request for help from staff was not being heard and therefore he felt he had to hit others back to *"show him that he can't mess with me"*. Steve also tended to rely on others to cope with difficult situations. He struggled to identify any useful coping strategies that he could utilise in these situations. For this reason, this EWS-R plan was constructed as primarily a team-based plan in contrast to Rakeem's shown in Table 5.1 earlier.

Stage 4: Feeding Back to the Wider MDT

Once the EWS-R plan was agreed, the findings were fed back to the larger team to gain consensus and implement the plan. This was done during handover and during MDT or ward rounds. The plan was entered into the clinical notes.

Stage 5: Monitoring and Reviewing

In order to monitor the effectiveness of the EWS-R, the team was encouraged to document whenever Steve became physically aggressive using the CBRS-P. Any changes would then be used to update his EWS-R plan.

Table 5.2 Steve's EWS-R Plan for Physical Violence Towards Others (e.g. punching, hitting)

	Signs Steve may show before engaging in this behaviour	How Steve normally behaves	How Steve behaves prior to the risk behaviour occurring	Action: What to do to help Steve
Earliest Signs	1 Making repeated requests (for leave, high-energy drinks and snacks) (contextual sign)	Normally Steve presents as quite calm and chatty at times. He is not particularly demanding.	Steve can start to swear and make derogatory and racists remarks if he feels his requests are denied, if he feels frustrated, targeted, undermined or ashamed.	To remind Steve that despite him feeling upset it is not okay to swear and encourage him to refrain. If unsuccessful staff to encourage Steve to go to his room and practice his TIPP skills. When calm, for staff to sit with Steve and talk about recent outburst.
	2 Consuming lots of energy drinks (visual sign)	Due to Steve having diabetes and being overweight, Steve has been trying to lose weight and limits himself to drinking one energy drink per day.	Consuming frequent energy drinks. Highly talkative pacing the unit and repeatedly approaching staff. Makes derogatory comments towards staff and expresses paranoid ideas that staff and peers don't like him.	Staff to provide reassurance and encourage him to relax. Staff to suggest activities he enjoys and may calm him down (e.g. listen to his music, practice TIPPS skills). Nurse in charge is to liaise with Steve and his family and remind them how energy drinks are affecting Steve's mood and behaviour.
Middle Signs	3 Non-compliance with medication (contextual and visual sign)	Steve will comply with his medication regime although he denies having any mental illness. Complains about side effects.	Challenges his medication and may become non-compliant. Responding to voices, TV and radio talking to him and commenting on his actions) – talking back to them out loud.	Nurse in Charge is to support Steve to understand the rational and importance of taking his medication. Provide leaflets (which Steve likes) about his medication, which he can take away and read in his own time. If his non-compliance continues, then to discuss at MDT or ward round about how to manage his non-compliance. The Responsible Clinician (RC) may also need to be informed, should his medication need reviewing.

(Continued)

Table 5.2 (Continued)

	Signs Steve may show before engaging in this behaviour	How Steve normally behaves	How Steve behaves prior to the risk behaviour occurring	Action: What to do to help Steve
Late Signs	4 Persecutory delusions (verbal and visual signs)	Steve will always exhibit a low-level paranoia but will engage in conversations with staff coherently. He can be polite and friendly but always has a short temper and is quick to anger.	Express frequent persecutory delusions (which may be a result of cannabis use): e.g. others are out to get him for his past misdeeds. Believing staff are in league with past bullies and enemies. Confronts staff asking them how they know X and how much are they getting paid.	Offer one-to-one time to listen to his concerns in a calm space and suspend disbelief. Review medication needs. Offer PRN if required (e.g. if he becomes increasingly angry and upset) Offer meaningful activities (e.g. Xbox, reading newspapers, playing cards, trivia quiz cards) to distract him and help to maintain trust.
	5 Verbal abuse (verbal sign)	Steve may initiate conversations and greet staff politely and ask about their well-being. His demeanour looks relaxed, while he is sitting on the sofa watching TV or listening to his music.	Is racially abusive and makes derogatory remarks (calling staff "bitches") Becomes intrusive i.e. repeatedly asks the same questions to meet his needs (e.g. request for unescorted leave) Makes inappropriate sexual comments. Make physical threats (e.g. will punch you in staff in the face). Scowls at staff and peers. Has frequent altercations with peers.	Continue to offer a 1:1 time in a quiet place, where Steve can safely express his distress. Provide Steve with reassurance that he is safe but acknowledge his concerns. Remind Steve of boundaries and reinforce the consequences of his behaviour with regard to his care plans and home leave. The Responsible Clinician (RC) would need to be informed, should his medication need reviewing.

TIPP: Temperature, Intense exercise, Paced breathing, Progressive muscle relaxation.

Summary

In this chapter, we have outlined key methods for monitoring and managing psychotic relapse and acute risk. Our approach is flexible and aimed at meeting the case-specific and changing needs of the service user. We utilise a number of tools to engage the service user and family where possible alongside utilising the resources and strengths of the MDT. EWS-R can help to predict risk. However, this is likely to be useful only if utilised to implement a care plan that is consistently delivered. EWS-R moreover helps the team to think about future placements and situations and how the individual can manage these safely.

Key to both approaches is having a clear and operationally defined target behaviour agreed upon from the beginning. As with all formulations in SAFE, these should be regularly reviewed and updated with additional information incorporated as it emerges.

It is important to consider creative ways of building relationships with service users who can be hard to reach such as the example in the chapter of using a group-based early warning signs programme to reduce shame and stigma and improve understanding of idiosyncratic relapse signatures and plans. Ultimately, the aim is to enable recovery and for service users to be able to recognise and manage their own early warning signs. Difficulties in achieving these may be some of the most important barriers to overcome.

Chapter 6

CARM Revisited

Introduction

The SAFE approach utilises a variety of formulations with the aim of increasing team empathy and compassion towards service users and providing evidence-based, psychologically informed care. The approach to assessment, formulation and intervention is key, and perhaps none more so in evidence when developing risk management plans. This chapter focuses on the use of the CARM (Meaden & Hacker, 2010) shared formulation and describes an approach built on the foundations of applied behavioural science – in particular, functional assessment and cognitive therapy for psychosis. This chapter advances some of the core principles underpinning CARM formulations and considers the processes involved in developing an understanding of problematic and risk behaviours that can be used to develop intervention and management plans. Chapters 7 and 9 build on this chapter, describing how we can use CARM formulations to develop care plans and need-adapted interventions.

Cognitive Approach to Risk Management

As has been discussed in previous chapters, the SAFE approach focuses attention on problematic behaviour and distress and how these serve as barriers to recovery amongst people who are experiencing psychosis, who are hard to reach and have complex behavioural needs. As such, one of the key targets for intervention is behaviour, and understanding the presence or absence of behaviour is a key task. CARM takes principles from behavioural science and cognitive therapy theory and integrates these to understand and explain problematic behaviours. Two CARM templates are provided in Appendices 2 and 3 – one each for "active" behaviours and "passive" behaviours. The core components include a specific problematic (or target) behaviour itself, behavioural reinforcements, immediate triggers to the behaviour, the setting events that led up to the presentation of the behaviour and the vulnerability factors that predispose the person to act in the way that they do. In addition to this, the CARM formulation also incorporates the early warning signs of the behaviour in question (see Chapter 5), as this is

DOI: 10.4324/9781003082811-7

often key in developing treatment plans and provides the basis for TBCT (see Chapter 8).

Meaden and Hacker (2010) originally articulated the limitations of other approaches to problematic behaviour in detail. Drawing on previous approaches from cognitive-behavioural therapy theory (Haddock et al., 2004, 2009) and behavioural models (Beer, 2006; Emerson, 2001), CARM integrates these into a functional model. Perhaps, most importantly, CARM redefines the target of intervention away from persistent symptoms and cognitive appraisals. These are conceptualised as vulnerability factors and unlikely to be responsive to direct intervention. The CARM formulation framework is specifically designed to enable staff within an MDT to develop a better understanding of how idiosyncratic, cognitive and behavioural factors interact within the service user's current social context to lead to problematic behaviours. It provides the team with multiple points for intervention with the aim of addressing behaviours early. CARM formulations are most effectively deployed when used to understand behaviours that are currently present and can be observed. The various components of the behaviour, experience and cognition can then be assessed in vivo, the CARM formulation developed with this information, interventions designed and implemented, the behaviour reassessed, and if necessary, the CARM formulation adapted in light of the new information. CARM formulations can be used with historical behaviours, but due to the need to consider the detail of the topography of the behaviour, such as its form, absence, presence and key triggers, a detailed amount of information is required to be able to populate the formulation and make this as accurate as possible. This can make it less useful for low-frequency historical behaviours, and the service user may be better served by other risk assessment schemes and formulations (see Chapter 4). Critical to the CARM formulation is being clear on the problematic behaviour – both the topography (the form of the behaviour) and whether it is hypothesised that there may be single or multiple functions to the behaviour.

Importance of Operationalising the Definition

The core principle behind our approach to formulation is to understand the function (or functions) of the behaviour – in other words, developing a set of hypotheses, derived from evidence (practice-based and research-based) about why the person is behaving in the way they are so that these can be used to inform attempts to change or manage that behaviour. It is not unusual to have multiple CARM formulations for a given individual. Consider for example the notion of violence or aggression – such terms are behaviourally vague as they could equally include behaviours such as shouting at others, attacking others with a weapon or breaking the property of others. It is critical here to understand what behaviours are being referred to when the formulation is first developed and to be clear what these look like. We find that it is helpful to ask ourselves and the team the question: would I know it from this description if I saw it? Once we have a clear idea of the kinds of behaviour being referred to, we can then embark on trying to understand the function.

Form and Function

Once we know the form that behaviour takes, we can start to develop hypotheses regarding the possible function it serves. Understanding the function of a behaviour can be used to improve outcomes for the service user, such as developing empathy amongst the staff team and understanding and managing the factors underpinning the presentation of the need met by the behaviour. Most importantly, care plans can be devised to help the person meet the function in a more appropriate way such as asking for help or being appropriately assertive. Often, when asked to describe a problem behaviour, teams will respond with a description that is vague and not effectively operationalised (e.g. aggression) or by suggesting its function (e.g. attention-seeking). The task in both instances is to clarify the form the behaviour takes.

Service users will often present with a variety of challenging and risk behaviours (Meaden et al., 2014), and it is possible that the function of each behaviour is the same and the same factors contribute to the presence of all these behaviours.

Case Illustration: Otis

Otis presents with risk behaviours which are interlinked and appear to meet the same function. In such formulations, some risk behaviours may be viewed as early warning signs for the target behaviour.

Target Behaviour (Throwing Objects at Others)

Otis insults staff calling them "dickhead" and issuing threats: "I will smash your head in, Miss"; "I'll fucking stab the lot of you", when his needs are not being met or when he feels he is being treated unfairly. He feels belittled and powerless at these times and tries to establish his authority by verbally insulting or intimidating staff. Also, he struggles to manage his emotions in a healthy way. When met with persistent refusal to meet his needs, Otis can quickly become highly agitated and aroused and can lash out and throw objects as a way to express his frustrations and to manage his intolerable emotions. When staff calmly intervene to move him to a safe place, he will attempt to hurt himself by headbutting the wall.

Otis has acquired various diagnosis from frontal lobe brain injury, Tourette's Syndrome and Attention Deficit Hyperactivity Disorder (ADHD) (all during childhood) to paranoid schizophrenia. Often, his behaviour is interpreted as poor impulse control due to neurological factors or being paranoid. Otis however shows no current active symptoms of psychosis. He is generally suspicious of others, which can be seen in the context of an abusive and neglected upbringing.

Careful observation shows that Otis will throw the least harmful objects available, indicating that he possesses a degree of control and that this may be a form of protest behaviour rather an intent to cause significant harm. When people do not back down, self-harm is the next chain of behaviour. Finally, Otis will try to intimidate the staff and make physical gestures as if he is going to swing a punch at them or headbutt them. However, he does not make actual physical contact with the staff.

In Otis's case, all of his behaviours function to get immediate needs met. They escalate according to the response of others, culminating in self-harm only when his efforts to assault others are prevented.

However, it may be that each behaviour serves different functions for the person – such as emotional expression (shouting), acting on delusional threat (use of a weapon), punishing others for perceived misdeeds (breaking property). Such aspects of the behaviour should be considered and discussed at the start of the process and ideally with the involvement of the service user and their loved ones – many of whom will have useful insights into the lived world of the person and their ways of making sense. When developing our understanding of the function of the behaviour, we can look to some of the principles that underpin functional assessment of problematic behaviour.

Principles of Functional Assessment

Hanley (2012) outlines three key types of functional assessment. The first kind is an indirect assessment, which involves the use of rating scales, interviews, questionnaires, etc. but does not include a direct observation of the behaviour in question. This might include clinician-rated outcome measures and self-report scales. The second kind of assessment is a descriptive assessment where there is direct observation of the behaviour but without any attempt to modify the conditions or context the behaviour appears in. This includes Antecedent-Behaviour-Consequence (the behavioural ABC; not to be confused with the cognitive ABC model) charts that many clinicians are familiar with. The third kind of assessment is a functional analysis, which involves direct observation of the problematic behaviour and an attempt to modify the environmental context to observe the impact on the behaviour. This last kind is used to explore potential causal links between environmental factors and the problematic behaviour.

In our experience, most functional risk assessments within complex and enduring mental health settings fall into the former two categories, as there is no attempt to experimentally manipulate the environment to observe the impact on the behaviour. While experimental paradigms are powerful techniques for establishing causal relationships, there are a variety of issues that limit the application of these in the settings where our service users are seen. The most obvious of these is the problem of how high-risk the behaviour is; it is simply not appropriate to manipulate potential variables if the operationalised behaviour is violent assault, as even a single occurrence of the behaviour is unacceptable. Another issue is that we may be called upon to assess and formulate a behaviour where factors associated with the behaviour are hidden from observable analyses or not open to manipulation (such as hallucinations, attitudes or delusional beliefs) and as such it is exceedingly difficult to develop effective behavioural analyses to experimentally establish their function. This means that although we may usefully borrow some of the principles from functional assessment, the formulations that we develop, including CARM, remain a collection of hypotheses that we must be open to revising and modifying in the face of disconfirmatory evidence. This serves to model a scientific approach to the team rather than jumping to conclusions by ourselves about the form and function of the behaviour.

Components of CARM

In this section, we discuss the different components of the CARM formulation and how these are employed in the SAFE process.

Reinforcers

Once we have identified the target risk behaviour and developed an operationalised definition of this, we can then turn to identifying and agreeing what factors may maintain this behaviour. If a behaviour is indeed dysfunctional, then we must establish what factors serve to reinforce and therefore maintain it. External reinforcers are arguably the most readily cited and observed (e.g. staff members avoid a service user when they are verbally threatened with violence). Internal reinforcers are, by contrast, the private events within the inner world of the individual but may be indirectly observable through external indicators (e.g. feelings of relief may be inferred from relaxing body posture, quietening voice, calming movements). Potential internal reinforcers include emotional states (e.g. reduction in anxiety, increasing happiness), psychotic symptoms (e.g. reduced delusional distress, increased positive voices) and cognitive states (e.g. increased perceived social rank, self-esteem, power). Potential external reinforcers include resources (e.g. cigarettes, food, money), social contact (e.g. friends, carers, staff) and environmental stimuli (e.g. noisy ward, preferred activities). Additionally, we can consider reinforcers across two broad areas – positive reinforcement (increased access to a desired stimulus that increases the likelihood of the behaviour) and negative reinforcement (the removal of an aversive stimulus that increases the likelihood of the behaviour) – see Cipani (2018) for a thorough consideration of these areas. A behaviour that increases our access to a desired outcome is likely to be repeated, while one that allows us to escape an aversive stimulus is also likely to be repeated. It is also worth bearing in mind that such functions can also be "direct" or "socially mediated" (Cipani, 2018). Direct or automatic reinforcement is where the person's behaviour leads to immediate access or removal of the stimulus (e.g. going to the kitchen to collect one of my biscuits; listening to music to drown out my critical voices). Socially mediated reinforcement is when the person's behaviour leads to access or removal of the stimulus through someone else (e.g. pestering another resident until they give me one of their biscuits; punching a staff member to prevent a feared discharge from hospital). It is our experience that many of our service users' behaviours may be maintained by socially mediated reinforcers, particularly where they are in restricted environments such as secure hospitals and their direct access to resources is limited.

Reinforcers are more likely to have their effects within particular (internal and external) circumstances, known as "establishing operations" (Keller & Schoenfeld, 1950), which increase the motivation for the problematic behaviour to occur (Cipani, 2018). For this reason, it is important to understand the factors that make the challenging behaviour more likely to occur in the first place – commonly known as antecedents. In the SAFE approach, we divide these across "triggers" and "setting events" (Carr et al., 1998), a distinction acknowledged in the literature on challenging behaviour (e.g. Simó-Pinatella et al., 2013) and one that makes targeting interventions more precise whilst also creating more points of intervention thus maximising opportunities to reduce the chances of the behaviour from occurring.

Triggers

Triggers are factors (internal and external to the person) that immediately precede the problematic or risk behaviour. They push the person into displaying the behaviour and are closely linked to reinforcing factors.

Case Illustration: Leam

Leam has been dwelling on derogatory auditory hallucinations that he believes come from another service user. The voices content makes him feel ashamed as they call him a "paedo". Leam has a history of sexual abuse and was subjected to child prostitution. He repeatedly shouts at his peer to stop the perceived persecution. The trigger that leads to the presence of behaviour in this example are feelings of shame. Reinforcers come in the form of the accused service user apologising to Leam (in order to get respite from Leam shouting at him). This has the effect for Leam of reducing his feelings of shame (a negative reinforcer).

Given the temporal proximity of triggers to the target behaviour, interventions that focus on triggers are likely to require preparatory work with either the service user in order to access potential internal triggers or the environment in order to access external triggers and to manage their presence. Once a trigger occurs, the likelihood of the behaviour following is increased – unless other moderating factors are present (e.g. the other service user getting up and leaving the communal area as soon as Leam walks in).

Setting Events

Setting events (both internal and external to the person) build the motivational state that increases the likelihood that the problematic behaviour will occur in the presence of relevant triggers. These are often harder to identify as they tend to be temporally distant from the trigger and behaviour. They are however no less important in establishing the function of the behaviour that follows and are often more likely to be targets for intervention. Time needs to be devoted to discussing and identifying them. Good quality observation may be needed to accurately identify and confirm them.

For Leam, internal setting events include dwelling on derogatory hallucinations and the beliefs about their origin (e.g. they come from another service user). External setting events may include news on the television about child abuse. These factors all increase the likelihood of the trigger (feelings of shame) and the subsequent shouting behaviour as an attempt to escape feelings of shame.

Using Setting Events to Derive EWS-R

Unlike triggers, setting events are less closely linked in time to the presence of the risk behaviour and can be good candidates for deriving EWS-R. These constitute the unique signs and patterns of behaviour, affect and cognition that reliably present prior to the defined outcome, in this case, the challenging or risk behaviour. There is consistent evidence for the utility of early warning signs as part of identifying early signs of relapse (see Chapter 5). We call these EWS-P in order to distinguish them from EWS-R, though they may be very similar in some cases. EWS-R constitute the observable (external) or reportable (internal) factors that are seen to precede the risk behaviour. These include operationalised (i.e. would we know it if we saw it?) versions of the antecedents with a strong emphasis on the setting events, given that these are more distally related to the risk behaviour and therefore offer more opportunity for intervention.

In Leam's case, EWS-R can be readily observed in his demeanour: his head hangs down and he avoids eye contact. He is also more irritable in his mood and very sensitive to any perceived criticism.

EWS-R can be used to identify potentially problematic establishing operations, and interventions can then be targeted to reduce the likelihood of the behaviour. In this sense, EWS-R can integrate well with PBS plans (Allen et al., 2005) and can be used to identify the need to divert people away from aversive establishing operations or reinforcers (i.e. EWS-R could include "amber" behaviours from the PBS system).

Vulnerability Factors

Vulnerability factors are predisposing factors that include both static risk factors (such as age, cohort, gender, personality traits) and longer-term dynamic-stable risk factors (e.g. auditory hallucinations, persecutory delusions, poor insight into mental health needs, attitudes supportive of instrumental violence, neurological and developmental factors). These are considered as the context within which the individual is sensitive to appraising internal and external events in ways which lead to problem behaviours.

Case Illustration: Leam

As well as shouting at peers, Leam also presents with more hostile assaultive behaviours: punching and grabbing staff by their hair. Leam learnt from an early age that others would exploit him whilst apparently being in a caring role. He was prostituted by his mother who was herself a sex worker. Certain staff are viewed with hostility by Leam (which is further supported by critical voices) if he perceives they look like his mother or know him from the past. When they are on shift (external setting event) and Leam is approached by them (external trigger) he fears that they intend to abuse him (internal trigger) and he attacks them. Over time, many members of the staff keep away from Leam whenever possible (acting as a negative reinforcer – reduced distress and shame).

Case Study: Timothy

Timothy is a 30-year-old male, who has been in touch with mental health services since his first episode of psychosis when he was 19 years old. Timothy is currently resident at a Community Rehabilitation Unit (CRU) following transfer from a High Dependency Unit (HDU). The current inpatient admission has lasted several years involving various hospital stays and was precipitated by physical aggression towards family members following excessive alcohol and cocaine use. Timothy is detained under Section 3 of the Mental Health Act. He has successfully engaged in risk management work and is actively involved in implementing his risk management plan for violence. Timothy's MDT are happy for him to be discharged into a supported living placement. However, since transfer to the CRU Timothy has been making sexualised comments and asking questions of (predominantly) female staff (e.g. "Have you ever kissed a woman?", "Does your boyfriend hold your hand in public?"). The team are worried about this, particularly in the context of discharge planning. A CARM formulation for "active behaviours" was developed with Richard's involvement (see Figure 6.1).

It was hypothesised that the core function of the socially and sexually inappropriate questions from Timothy was to express a need for social connection and intimacy. Timothy had already discussed with

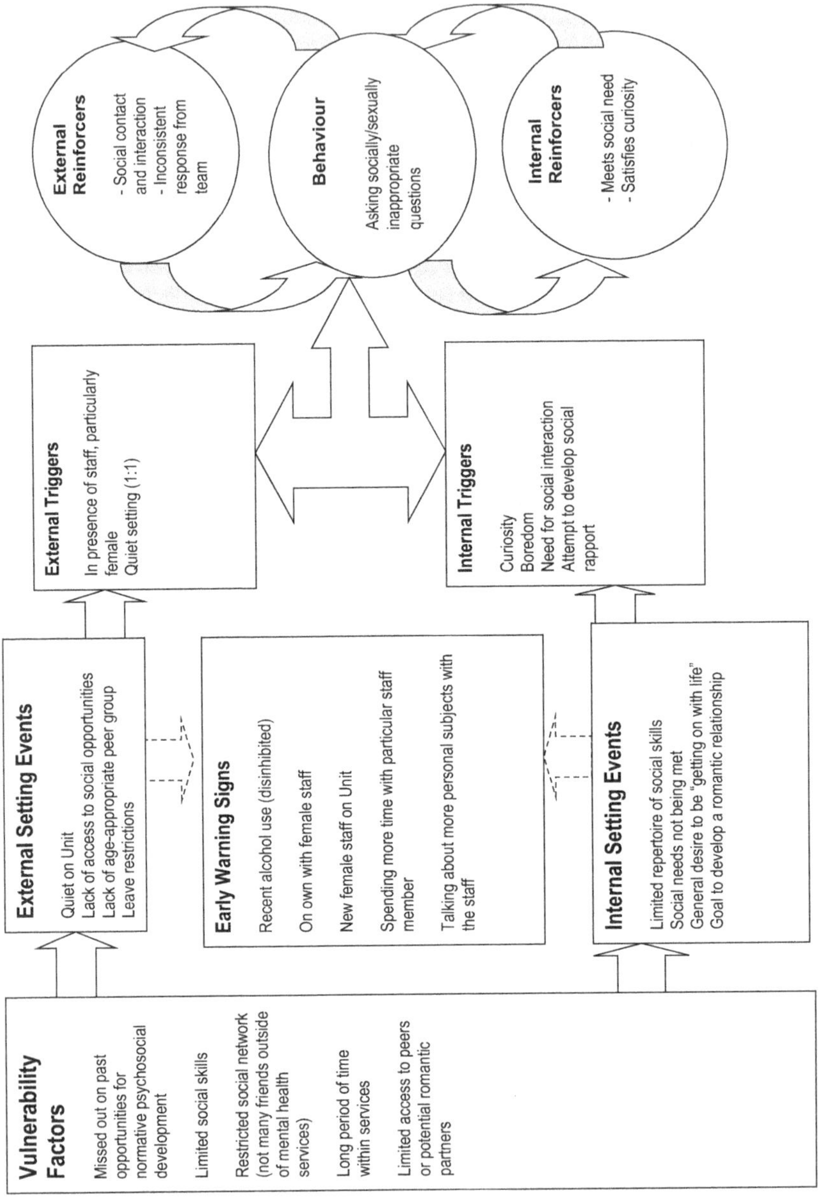

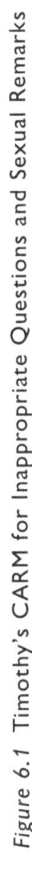

Vulnerability Factors

Missed out on past opportunities for normative psychosocial development

Limited social skills

Restricted social network (not many friends outside of mental health services)

Long period of time within services

Limited access to peers or potential romantic partners

External Setting Events

Quiet on Unit
Lack of access to social opportunities
Lack of age-appropriate peer group
Leave restrictions

Early Warning Signs

Recent alcohol use (disinhibited)

On own with female staff

New female staff on Unit

Spending more time with particular staff member

Talking about more personal subjects with the staff

Internal Setting Events

Limited repertoire of social skills
Social needs not being met
General desire to be "getting on with life"
Goal to develop a romantic relationship

External Triggers

In presence of staff, particularly female
Quiet setting (1:1)

Internal Triggers

Curiosity
Boredom
Need for social interaction
Attempt to develop social rapport

External Reinforcers

- Social contact and interaction
- Inconsistent response from team

Behaviour

Asking socially/sexually inappropriate questions

Internal Reinforcers

- Meets social need
- Satisfies curiosity

Figure 6.1 Timothy's CARM for Inappropriate Questions and Sexual Remarks

peers and staff that a key recovery aim for him was to "meet someone, have a family". Timothy had been involved in services, including inpatient admissions, from a young age (19), has had limited opportunities to develop his social skills in this area and experienced limited romantic and sexual opportunities. Timothy moreover had a very limited social network such that he had very few similar-age peers and none who were outside of the mental health services. As such, Timothy had very few opportunities to explore his sexuality or make any social connections with others. It was hypothesised that his attempts to do this were naturally more likely to occur with those he had access to (staff team) and that he was somewhat naïve and socially clumsy. This appeared more frequent when Timothy had been drinking alcohol – which appeared to have a disinhibitory effect. Within the staff team there were a range of responses to Timothy's questions – some staff perceived him as younger than his years and viewed his questions as genuine (albeit inappropriate) attempts to satisfy his curiosity, and they would sometimes answer his questions if they did not deem them too excessive a boundary transgression. Alternatively, other staff indicated that they viewed his comments or questions as wholly unacceptable and advocated a "zero-tolerance" approach, admonishing Timothy for such questions. This inconsistent approach in the team seemed to be contributing to Timothy's uncertainty regarding socially acceptable behaviour and this was underpinned by his limitations in his social skills, lack of experience and limited avenues to express his needs. The formulation was shared with Timothy in a narrative format. Timothy agreed with this.

A care plan was developed in agreement with Timothy for social skills training sessions with the unit psychologist, focussed on the development of social and psychosexual knowledge alongside social skill (see Fox & Harrop, 2015). To help practice skills and socialise Richard into the approach, joint sessions with the (male) psychologist and (female) occupational therapist were used. to provide a safe and boundaried forum for Timothy. Inappropriate questions and comments were redirected to the regular social skills training sessions. These sessions moved into the community to practise social skills in vivo, and Timothy was encouraged to start at an adult education centre to prepare for retaking his secondary education qualifications. This also offered him an opportunity to practise his skills and meet his social needs outside of mental health services.

Developments in Utilising CARM Formulations

Over the last ten years, we have continued to use CARM as both a stand-alone shared formulation and also increasingly integrating it into other risk frameworks. It has also become clearer which behaviours are best suited to a CARM formulation and where it needs adapting (Meaden & Fox, 2015).

Deciding on the Behaviour

Some behaviours are more suited to formulating with our CARM template. Most relevant are high-frequency active behaviours. These are often the most distressing for the team and therefore the ones they are most motivated to address. Addressing problem behaviours is a lengthy and time-consuming process; so, having motivated staff is vital. These behaviours are also the most observable and therefore easiest to gather information about. Other behaviours can be formulated using CARM, including what we originally termed behavioural deficits and now term "passive" behaviours (see Fox & Meaden, 2015); however, again, these work best when the behaviour is periodically present and absent, in order to gain information about the form of the behaviour and the establishing operations prior to its occurrence. In cases where an important behaviour is absent for long periods of time (e.g. not washing), it is difficult to develop an understanding of the setting events and triggers, as the behaviour is defined as problematic by its continual omission. In these cases, CARM may be less useful, and other forms of formulation may be better suited to the task, such as a narrative "descriptive" formulation or the cross-sectional cognitive ABC formulation.

CARM for Passive Behaviours

When considering the challenges associated with so-called "negative symptoms" of Schizophrenia, we have previously identified adaptations to the traditional CARM formulation that incorporate developments in cognitive theory (Fox & Meaden, 2015), particularly regarding negative expectancy appraisals (Rector et al., 2005). It has been argued that the amotivational state associated with negative symptoms is characterised by avolition and a reduction in appetitive drive (i.e. "wanting") with the consummatory drive ("liking") left intact (Foussias & Remington, 2010). Beck and colleagues suggest that beliefs indicative of low expectancies of pleasure, acceptance and achievement may explain lack of motivation to engage in goal-directed behaviour (Beck & Rector, 2005). If we expect to fail, then there is little drive to engage in a behaviour. Integrating this into the CARM approach, we begin by focusing on the MDT's views and understanding of the often puzzling and frustrating (for families, caregivers and staff) presentations usually collected under the umbrella of negative symptoms, such as poor self-care, social withdrawal, poor communication and lack of emotional expression. We now refer to these behaviours as "passive" in that they indicate a lack of action where typically action is expected. As noted in Chapter 1, some behaviours may appear to be passive behaviours: lying on the floor. However, when their function is examined more carefully, they may in fact constitute active behaviours. These are what we now term "active resistance" behaviours. Care must therefore be taken to ensure that we are utilising the correct CARM formulation for the problem. An active CARM formulation may be developed first to test out the function. Where behaviours are hypothesised to constitute passive behaviours more clearly, this terminology enables the team to better avoid the assumption that such behaviours (or lack of it) are driven by illness-related symptoms or that there is an internally driven deficit (the belief that one will fail, for example, is not accurately considered a "deficit").

The adaptations to CARM for passive behaviours can be seen in our template in Appendix 3. We have removed early warning signs, as passive behaviours are often present at a high frequency but also tend to present a lower immediate risk, which reduces the accuracy and practicality of such signs. Instead, the focus is on the identification of negative outcome appraisals or expectations of the service user. These can be pan-situational beliefs (generalised beliefs that apply across multiple situations) or in-situation inferences (specific expectations to the behaviour being formulated) and are the cognitive states (internal setting events) associated with negative affect and low motivation (internal triggers) for goal-directed behaviour. These provide the establishing operations for the reinforcement of behaviour that allows for the avoidance or escape of the negative cognitions and/or affective state. Important external setting events will be environments or behaviours of others that activate the negative outcome appraisals, such as the need to complete tasks or requests to participate. However, it is the completion of valued activities that is a key process through which negative appraisals and associated affect can be managed, as, given an intact consummatory reward system, it is (at least theoretically) possible for the person to gain a sense of achievement or pleasure from the activity. Repeated opportunities for the disconfirmation of negative outcome expectancies can therefore be offered as interventions. However, these will be successful only if the person makes a "leap of faith" and engages in an activity they expect to fail or not enjoy. Therapeutic optimism and the development of a strong therapeutic relationship grounded on trust, genuineness and unconditional positive regard are necessary pre-requisites for this type of intervention. This emphasises the importance of working collaboratively with service users and with the whole MDT (whose members may have established therapeutic relationships with service users).

Case Study: Sandra

Sandra is in her late fifties. She moved to a Long-Term Complex Care Unit (LCCU) 12 months ago following an acute relapse. Sandra has spent the last 30 years in and out of community placements and supported living flats, but these have all broken down: she will neglect her personal care and has been found "wandering" out in the street late at night. She is on the caseload of local community mental health team.

Sandra has a diagnosis of schizophrenia. Her father has passed away, and she has no contact with any family other than her elderly mother, with whom she used to live. Unfortunately, Sandra's mother had a fall and went to live in a residential home, leaving Sandra without somewhere to live, and this is when she first moved into a supported living placement, about ten years ago. At school, Sandra completed a handful of GCSEs; she has worked in some temporary factory placements but has not had a job in the last few years. She appears to struggle to remember things, possibly due to attentional difficulties and it has been noticed that, at times, Sandra appears distracted, as though listening to something. She denies hearing voices when asked; however, it is believed by the community team who have worked with her over the years that Sandra hears voices criticising her. On the LCCU, staff have occasionally heard Sandra seemingly talking to the voices under her breath. She usually forgets to take prescribed medication and requires help to remember this – with reminders she is concordant. She has diabetes, and this is managed through diet, which Sandra requires help with, as she does not believe that she has diabetes. The staff team report that they find social interactions with Sandra difficult as she makes little eye contact and does not engage in spontaneous speech, with the staff member taking the lead when chatting with her, which can be tiring over prolonged periods.

At the LCCU, Sandra usually appears quite dishevelled; she requires reminders to wash her hair, attend to personal care and to change her clothes. Without these reminders, she will wear the same clothes despite having lots of clothes in the wardrobe and will neglect her personal care. Sandra has indicated that she believes that other people think that she is "a failure", but when asked about this, she declines to discuss this.

Sandra requires prompts from others to make herself meals, preferring to eat takeaways. During meal preparation, she appears to know the steps of the skills but requires prompts and support to implement these. On some days, she will remain in her room in bed and requires regular prompts to get up to even make herself a drink. Sandra requires support to keep her room clean, seemingly getting "lost" when faced with the choices between different cleaning products and struggling to initiate the steps of the different skills (such as those involved in cleaning her shower or changing the duvet).

Each day, Sandra requires prompts to get up, make her breakfast with support from staff, take medication and then spends most of her time at the LCCU. Sandra has reported that she used to like visiting the local park to feed the ducks but has declined offers to visit. Sandra talks more to the team when outside the LCCU, for example when going to GP appointments with support from the staff. Sandra is under Section 3 of the Mental Health Act, as it is felt that she is a risk to herself (vulnerable to exploitation from others, chronic self-neglect, verbal aggression to others) and has indicated that she would not stay at the LCCU voluntarily. The staff report frustration with the lack of engagement from Sandra. Scores on the RRES reflect this, with "sometimes" commonly endorsed for items in the domains of "agreement with treatment and basic relationships" and "compliance with medication" and "rarely" or "never" for items in the "active participation" domain. Some staff suggest that perhaps this is "as good as it gets" for Sandra.

We can see how in Figure 6.2 the adapted CARM was used to develop a way of working with Sandra.

The case formulation team was assembled and the notes reviewed. We used the adapted CARM for passive behaviours to socialise the team into ways of understanding Sandra's difficulties. This was particularly important given her lack of discussion with the team about her inner world. The team had to rely (initially) on speculation based on past information as to what might be the key internal setting events. It was quickly identified that a potential reinforcing function of her passive behaviour (not engaging in core activity including self-care) was avoidance of failure. The key vulnerability factors were hypothesised as poor attention, concentration and memory (which sets her up to perform poorly on tasks). Sandra's limited range of hobbies were identified as a potential factor that reduced her range of opportunities for enjoyment, alongside avoidance of tasks that reduced the opportunity for the experience of success, pleasure and mastery of daily activities (such as self-care). Her tendency to believe that others thought badly of her was hypothesised to be based on her own self-critical beliefs, chronic self-focussed attention and/or poor "theory of mind". The potential negative outcome expectancies were also developed as a collection of

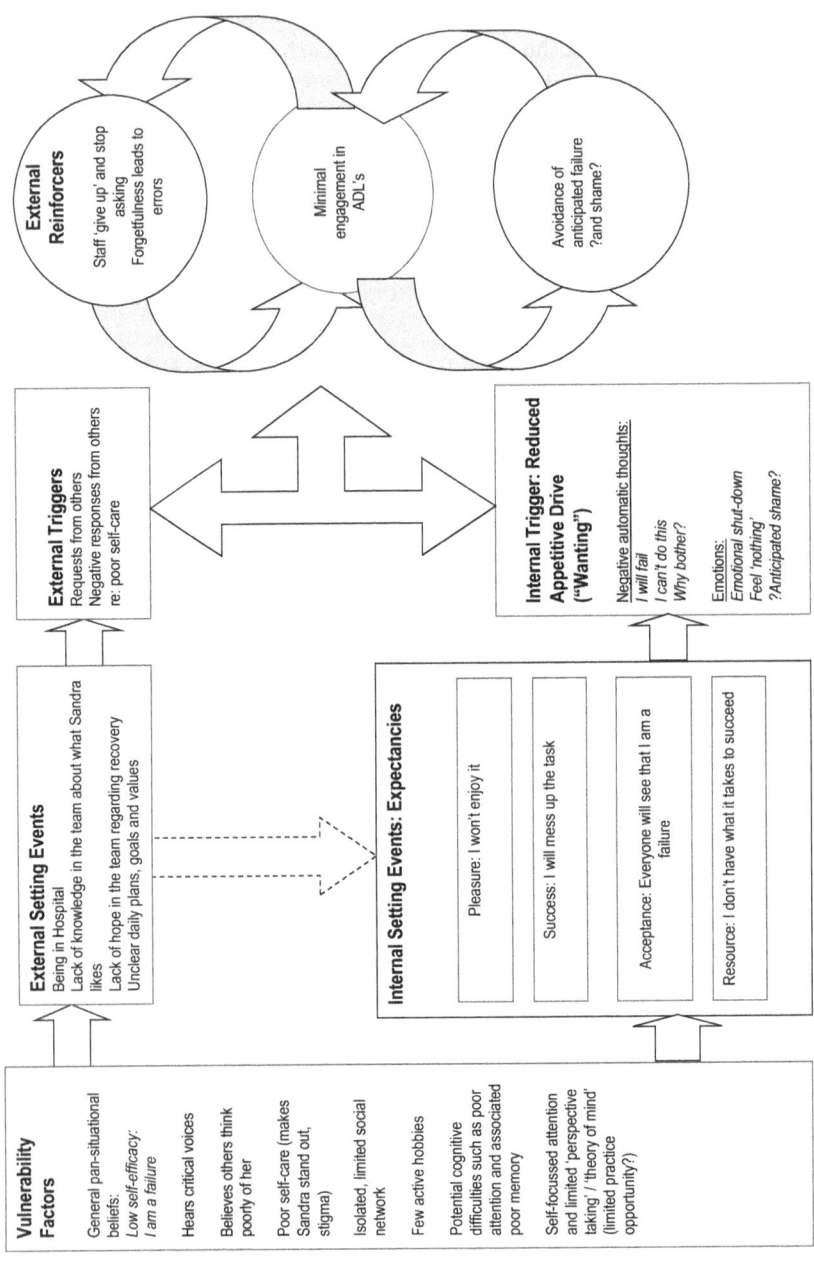

Figure 6.2 Sandra's CARM for Passive Behaviours

hypotheses in the formulation that were then explored through daily interactions with Sandra.

Two healthcare assistants with whom Sandra seemed able to discuss her experiences were key in helping to derive more accurate hypotheses regarding these expectancies. These were then explored through interactions with Sandra, and staff used reassurance to reduce the risk that daily task requests (such as to attend to self-care) were creating negative expectancies (e.g. "let's just have a go and see how things work out"). Positive feedback was given and attention drawn to Sandra's successes. Regular (monthly) supervision sessions were provided for the team to air any concerns or frustrations around the work in an effort to reduce negative feelings being expressed towards Sandra and inadvertently reinforce her fears of failure and criticism. Regular trips out with Sandra were scheduled at the same time every week so that she could become familiar with these, and Sandra was able to express her preference about where to go and what to do on these trips out (usually to a local park to feed the ducks and swans) to enhance her sense of agency and control.

The occupational therapist worked closely with Sandra and the rest of the team to identify short, focussed activities that she could take part in that had little chance of failure but that it was felt Sandra might enjoy based on experience (e.g. those based around animals, such as visits from therapy dogs). Care was also taken to develop tasks that could be completed without the need for extensive cognitive resources. Explicit yet sensitive positive feedback was given about the successes that Sandra had achieved when she did take part in a task (such as cooking). The team agreed to explicitly verbalise their thinking processes for Sandra, partly to reassure her that they were not thinking critically about her but also to overcome any hypothesised theory of mind or "perspective taking" difficulties Sandra might experience.

One key issue that was raised early on in team supervision was the difficulty in keeping Sandra's trips out scheduled on the LCCU activity planner. It was very easy for these to be "rescheduled" (or cancelled) due to more pressing concerns at the LCCU. Discussion with the team manager allowed the team to be reassured that Sandra's needs were of equally high priority and that resources would be made available to support these trips out. This helped to ensure that Sandra became familiar with the regular routine of the trips out and the team were implicitly reinforcing the message that she was of value (i.e. undermining any self-critical thoughts or voices). Of note at this point is that these strategies are underpinned by cognitive therapy principles but in a less explicit way. Consequently, Sandra's beliefs were not explicitly articulated to her nor alternatives presented. Rather, the emphasis was on gentle positive promotion to take part, with the aim of Sandra's changed behaviour promoting cognitive change in her expectancies.

Over time, the team started to develop a better idea of what was of value to Sandra and gained a better idea of her goals. It was then possible to translate these into more specific care plan goals. With subsequent increased hopefulness in the team for Sandra's recovery, the team was able to focus on daily interactions with her and how best to develop alternative expectancies for her (e.g. the phrase "you might enjoy it, but even if you don't, we can still have a go" modelling alternative healthy expectancies of pleasure, social acceptance and access to resource).

The Importance of Considering Internal Events

Compared to other areas of functional assessment, working with challenging behaviours in the context of psychosis requires a considerable focus on internal, private events that are, for the most part, unobservable. All three categories of internal events (setting, triggers, reinforcers) can be best identified and understood with involvement of the service user. However, service users can often be absent from the formulation process (e.g. due to poor relationships with the team, rejection of the need for any treatment) and in these cases, it is necessary to be clear that these aspects of the formulation are *hypotheses* that must be open to revision on the basis of new information. Nevertheless, it is our experience that such hypotheses can still be grounded in observable evidence such as physical indications of affective states (e.g. shaking when anxious), repeated claims from service users (e.g. expressed statements about intentions of others) or other patterns of cognition or behaviour (e.g. jumping to conclusions).

Knowledge of psychological theory is crucial in being able to develop hypotheses about possible internal events and how these may link to external (observable or social) factors. For example, we have found that social rank theory as applied to the experiences of psychosis (Wood & Irons, 2016) has been very useful in developing hypotheses regarding the processes through which service users may respond with strong emotions to seemingly innocuous staff requests. Advances in psychological theory and practice such as those seen in cognitive approaches to command hallucinations (Meaden et al., 2013) and sleep in psychosis (Waite et al., 2020) can be usefully drawn upon to illuminate internal processes that may be important to consider, including how such factors may interact. This is considered further in Chapter 9.

Order and Process of Collecting the Information

Our approach to CARM will always start with a clear definition and operationalisation of the behaviour. This is key to understanding the level of risk posed and to whom (e.g. service user themselves, family, care staff) and allows us to prioritise the behaviours for formulation should there be several types. An important consideration here is the function of the behaviour (e.g. cutting self with broken glass) and whether two behaviours that look similar may be underpinned by different functions (e.g. escape from aversive affective states, communicating distress to caregivers) – in which case it may be helpful to develop two different

CARM formulations, where the different factors that contribute to each pathway can be carefully considered.

Our experience suggests that it is often most helpful to move backwards from right to left through the CARM templates. We turn next to identification of the triggers, setting events and vulnerability factors, before considering reinforcers in light of these discoveries. Often, reinforcers can be fully formulated only once the establishing operations (i.e. the setting events and triggers) have been identified; so for this reason, they can usefully be left until the end. In practice, there is often a need to revisit components once other areas are illuminated.

Often, the people who have most access to information needed to best describe the behaviours and factors that are most relevant are staff who work with service users regularly such as healthcare assistants and nursing staff. Family and service users can also usefully be involved in helping to develop the CARM formulation. Involvement of the full MDT is always recommended as this is likely to best capture the perspectives of the team and be perceived as something plausible that can lead to meaningful interventions. Furthermore, this allows for the use of the CARM formulation in testing and modifying unhelpful assumptions and attitudes in the team: TBCT.

We propose that the team's beliefs should be viewed as legitimate intervention targets where they are associated with unhelpful responses that are incompatible with effective recovery-oriented interventions. In essence, challenging behaviours from service users can act as triggers for unhelpful assumptions about the nature and cause of these behaviours (e.g. that behaviour is deliberately manipulative) which leads to distress in the staff team and aversive care responses (e.g. avoidance, exclusion). Attitudinal changes can be achieved either explicitly through formal disputation processes or implicitly through providing a parsimonious explanation for service user behaviour that leads to more pragmatic interventions (see Fox & Meaden, 2015; Meaden et al., 2015). Either way, the focus is on realigning the team's beliefs such that the service user's behaviour no longer acts as an activating event that triggers assumptions associated with aversive care responses such as avoidance, exclusion or restraint. In our experience, completing the CARM formulation as a team is an ideal opportunity to identify such unhelpful beliefs and provide a more evidence-based and testable alternative (see Figure 6.3).

Identifying Factors for CARM Formulation

Behavioural recording sheets based on the behavioural ABC are a useful tool for developing an understanding of situation-specific factors that might contribute to the presence (or absence) of a behaviour. They also serve as a useful test for staff motivation. Given the emphasis on internal, unobservable factors, and the need to consider the wider context of the behaviours (vulnerability factors), other assessment methods will also likely be needed. Utilising the START as

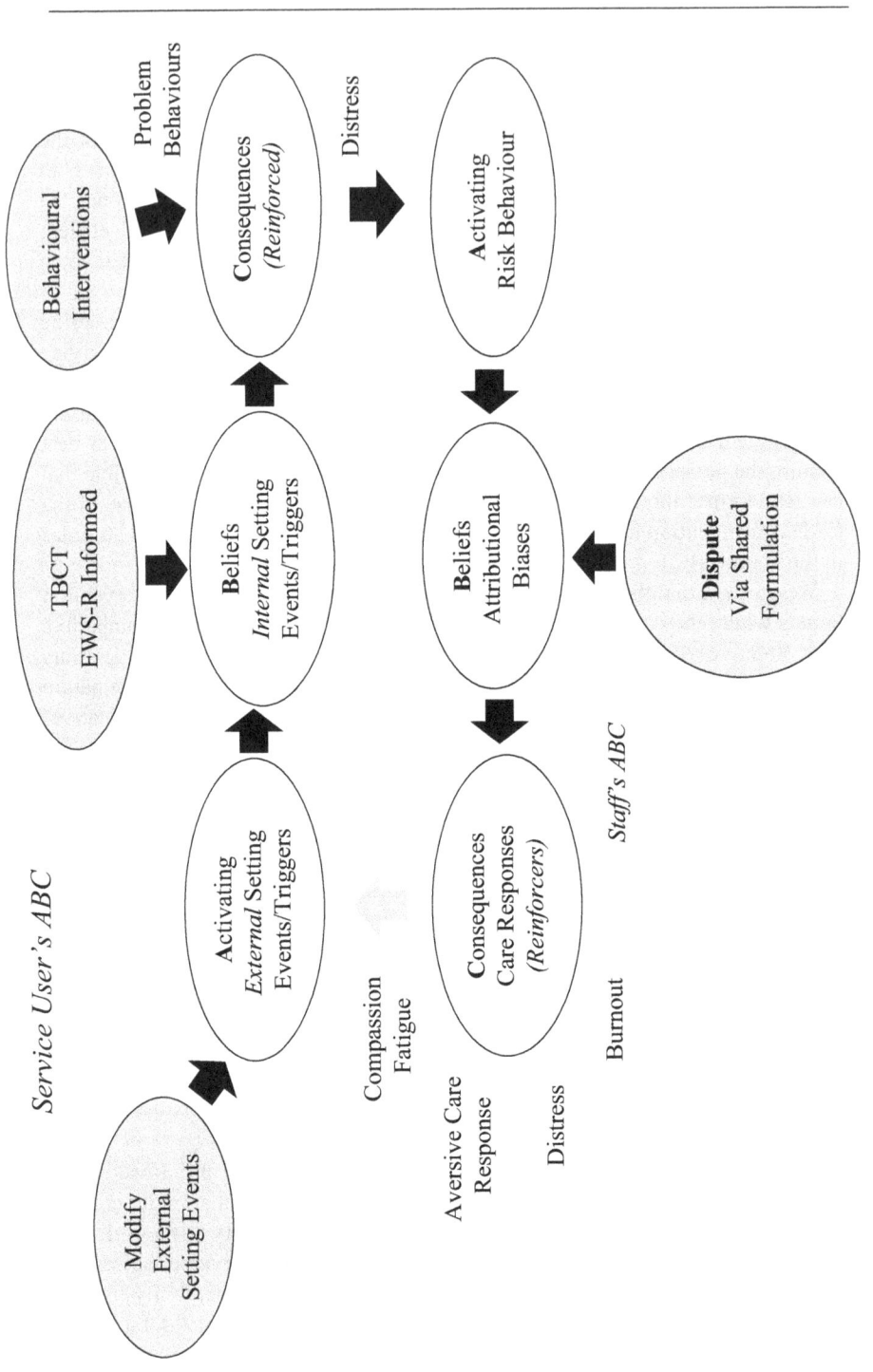

described in Chapter 4, we are able to identify likely dynamic factors that may provide establishing operations (e.g. negative affect, persecutory beliefs, poor social skill) for the reinforcing functions of risk behaviour. The START incident subscales are an additional aspect that we find useful for categorising a selection of risk behaviours and identifying those which will benefit from a CARM formulation. This provides fertile ground for the identification of problematic behaviour and the associated factors that can be subsequently incorporated into the CARM formulation. Often, the same factors will be incorporated into multiple CARM formulations.

Case Illustration: Carl

Carl has delusional beliefs about being poisoned through the drinking water. The same factors that help us understand his tendency to dismantle the taps and flood his room (delusional beliefs that staff are poisoning his water, anxiety about being poisoned) are also instrumental in understanding his tendency to shout violently at the unit staff (delusional beliefs that staff are poisoning the water, anger about being poisoned).

Should a factor in the formulation be identified as particularly significant, then this can be flagged as either an EWS-R of increasing risk (vulnerability) or a protective factor (strengths). Once identified, such signs and protective factors can be used to develop care plan targets, such as ways to enhance strengths or ways to manage risks.

Summary

In this chapter, we have described the CARM structure alongside the principles that underpin it. Also, we have outlined how we have refined our understanding and application of CARM through our practice and recent developments in psychological knowledge. It remains a team-based approach to understanding and managing problem behaviour and risk, and whilst time-consuming, we believe that the complexity of the needs of our service users merit such an approach. One of the strengths of the CARM is that interventions can have multiple potential targets (i.e. setting events, triggers, reinforcing factors), and these are considered further in our intervention chapters.

Chapter 7

Planning and Delivering Behavioural Interventions in SAFE

Introduction

In their previous work, Meaden & Hacker (2010) proposed a SMART methodology (Small, Measurable, Achievable, Relevant and Time-limited) for care planning utilising Goal Attainment Scaling Tool or GAST (Kiresuk et al., 1994) to specify the step to achieve each care plan goals. Over the last ten years while working in settings for those who are hard to reach and treat, we have found this approach to be too complex for most practitioners. It requires clinicians to turn presenting problems on their head and move away from conceptualising care plan goals in broad terms (e.g. improve personal hygiene) and to think very specifically and behaviourally about the problem. Care plan goals are turned into very concise goals and steps. A brief example might be the goal of washing one's hair at least twice a week; washing hair less than weekly would be at one end of the scale (0) and washing hair using shampoo twice weekly would be at the other end (5). This has proved too time-consuming for clinicians and is not in keeping with the often predominant psychiatric model in services which views problems at the broader symptom and syndrome level. A second significant barrier has been the clinical information system used. SMART and GAST were problematic in terms of how they could be both recorded and how outcome data could be generated, collated and reported. We achieved this in only one inpatient unit (the second authors) and in no community teams. Alongside this, there has been a growing interest in adopting PBS (DOH, 2014 and Skills for Care & Skills for Health, 2014). We found this fitted well with SAFE and appeared to be increasingly widely adopted elsewhere.

In this chapter, we describe our approach to incorporating PBS plans into services where SAFE is most relevant. It is a crucial step in the SAFE process where shared understandings are translated into care plans to support the delivery of SAFE interventions. We provide examples of how to implement this, highlight the difficulties and illustrate the process with relevant case examples.

DOI: 10.4324/9781003082811-8

What We Mean by Challenging and Risk Behaviour

In Chapter 1, we outlined the critical differences between challenging or problematic behaviour and risk behaviour, the latter being implicated in harm. Agreeing to what should be the treatment target and, by inference, the care plan goal can be an extremely complex issue. Those working with the person will often share different views on what is or is not challenging and how much this behaviour constitutes a risk to others. The function the behaviour serves for the individual is relevant but also the extent to which it impedes recovery or creates a barrier to social participation. A key question to ask is: "How feasible it is to address the behaviour given the current staffing levels, staff skill and type of environment (e.g. locked, open or community)". A further consideration is how much others can tolerate the behaviour exhibited. Our revised approach to categorising behaviours as active and passive helps to socialise others to avoid stating the function of the behaviour when it is described (which happens often automatically and implicitly). A familiar example would be describing a behaviour as "attention seeking" or "avoidance" which tells us nothing about the actual behaviour being exhibited (i.e. what does the person actually do?). We frequently ask, "would I know it if I saw it?" questions. Consequently, we ask for an explicit description: punching another resident in the face with a fist. Classification also helps us to categorise behaviours early on that are related to harm (risk behaviours) versus those that are challenging or labelled as problematic. This helps to prioritise care planning. Challenging behaviours can be ignored to reduce the possibility of reinforcing them whereas risk behaviours likely to lead to harm clearly cannot. Active behaviours are best suited to PBS planning.

An Overview of PBS

PBS plans underpin a person-centred, values-led approach to promoting behavioural change in people who challenge (Allen, 2020; BPS, 2018; Gore et al., 2013). This non-aversive behavioural model was first advocated by LaVigna and Donnellan (1986) and Horner et al. (1990) in their work establishing the principles of PBS. These are based on the principles of Social Role Valorisation (Wolfesnsberger, 1983), a dynamic set of ideas for making positive change in the lives of people disadvantaged because of their status in society and upon operant learning theory as first proposed by Skinner (1971). Put simply, challenging behaviour is maintained by the consequences that follow it and thus serves a function for that person. However, unlike meeting one's needs in a helpful or socially accepted way, the behaviour adopted can become a problem in itself (e.g. shouting to obtain attention, lying on the floor to avoid an activity). The aim therefore is to try to enable the person to meet their needs in more socially acceptable ways by modifying others' responses. Behaviourally based approaches have a long experimental and clinical research evidence base though they have until more recently largely fallen out of favour for the treatment of psychosis since the era of token economies (Ayllon & Azrin, 1968). PBS has brought behavioural approaches up to date and allowed for a more individualised and person-centred approach. In SAFE, the focus is always about reducing barriers to recovery. PBS-based interventions are consequently well suited as they aim to increase quality of life and decrease problem behaviour by teaching new skills to enhance the individual's behavioural repertoire to more socially appropriate ways of responding.

PBS emphasises the understanding of the behaviour from the person's point of view and their recovery goals. Its compatibility with SAFE is further supported by its use of functional analysis and assessments that culminate in an idiosyncratic formulation-based support plan. PBS utilises a broad range of theoretically informed interventions and approaches with the view to reducing the frequency of the challenging behaviour. Accordingly, TBCT can also be readily incorporated into PBS plans.

Characteristics of PBS

Horner et al. (1990) have defined the characteristics of PBS as follows.

1 It is values-led, in that the goal of behavioural strategies is to achieve enhanced community presence, choice, personal competence, respect and community participation, rather than simply behavioural change in isolation.
2 It is based on an understanding of why, when and how behaviours happen and what purposes they serve (via the use of functional analysis).
3 It focuses on altering triggers for behaviour in order to reduce the likelihood that the behaviour will occur.
4 It uses skill teaching as a central intervention, as lack of critical skills is often a key contributory factor in the development of behavioural challenges.
5 It uses changes in quality of life as both an intervention and an outcome measure.
6 It achieves reductions in challenging behaviour as a side effect of the aforementioned.
7 It has a long-term focus, as challenging behaviours are often of a long-term nature and successful interventions therefore need to be maintained over prolonged periods.
8 It has a multi-component focus, reflecting the facts that challenging behaviours often have multiple determinants and that service users typically display multiple forms.
9 It reduces or eliminates the use of punishment approaches.
10 It includes both proactive strategies for changing behaviour and reactive strategies for managing behaviour when it occurs, since even the most effective change strategies may not completely eliminate risk behaviours from behavioural repertoires.

Using PBS Principles in Hard-to-Reach-and-Treat Populations

The Royal College of Psychiatrists (2009) report service users accessing reha- bilitation services are probably one of the most complex and neglected groups a professional can work with. They state that this population is hard to prioritise in terms of care planning. Whilst PBS has its origins in working with service users with a primary learning disability (Allen, 2020; BPS, 2018; Gore et al., 2013), we see no reason why this approach cannot be used effectively in the population that SAFE was first developed for. Indeed, recent studies show the effectiveness of PBS in forensic mental health settings (e.g. Davies et al., 2019; Tolisano et al., 2017).

Constructing a PBS Plan

Having completed a START, CARM and a narrative static-dynamic formulation for each risk behaviour, the MDT are supported to agree which behaviour may be a useful initial focus for a PBS plan. As noted previously, active behaviours are usually most appropriate for PBS plans. Care should be given to consider the ability of the MDT and the suitability of the physical environment for safely managing the behaviour whilst attempting to modify them through a combination of EWS-R interventions, TBCT and behavioural (reinforcement-based) modifica- tion techniques. A useful framework to consider is the Risk, Needs, Responsivity Model (RNR), developed by Andrews et al. (1990) which has been an influential early model for the assessment and treatment of offenders.

Principle 1: Risk

- Is the intervention appropriate for the individual's level of risk?
- High Risk = higher levels of intervention (dose and intensity)
- Low Risk = low dose/intensity

Principle 2: Need

- Are the intervention targets matched to the individual's areas of criminogenic need?

Principle 3: Responsivity

- Is the individual *able to respond* to the intervention?
- Intervention should be provided in a way which is responsive to the indi- vidual's learning style, ability, strengths;
- Should also consider *barriers*, seek change through *reinforcement* and *problem-solving*;

- The relationship between the service user and the staff member should be – warm, respectful, built on a collaborative working alliance.

Stage 1: Operationally Defining the Target Behaviour (Red Behaviour)

The Challenging Behaviour Foundation (2014) is adopted in the development of a PBS plan. The first step is to arrive at a clear operational description. A traffic light system to categorise behaviour into clear care plan goals is as follows.

> *Red Behaviours:* constitute the problem behaviours and target of intervention. The so-called reactive strategies adopting a least restrictive practice approach are devised as part of a step-by-step plan to manage the behaviour and reduce the risk.
>
> *Amber Behaviours:* constitute our EWS-R. Strategies here aim to de-escalate the situation before the target behaviour occurs.
>
> *Green Behaviours:* are the alternative appropriate behaviours which are desired, for example asking for help rather than ordering the nurse to do something. Proactive strategies are designed to meet the person's needs without them needing to rely on challenging behaviours. This part of the plan should include any strategies that are aimed at reducing the chances that the behaviour will occur and should focus on all aspects of the person's life including keeping healthy and fit (as opposed to just focusing on the challenging behaviour). When exhibited a green behaviour, the service user is positively praised thus positively reinforcing this behaviour and increasing the likelihood of the behaviour occurring again.
>
> *Blue Strategies:* are employed after any incidents of the target behaviour occurring. They aim to help the service user remain calm and stable and thereby avoid another escalation of the behaviour. This can include giving the service user space, providing medical assistance if required, helping them to engage in a distracting activity or moving to a different calm space or room.

Stage 2: Clarifying the Person's Recovery Goals

As a next step, we draw on the findings from the SLF participation domain and the RGPI to clarify what recovery goals the person has and how the *Red Behaviour* acts as a barrier to achieving these. Also, we can refer to the narrative CARM and static-dynamic formulations for this behaviour.

Stage 3: Ensuring Red Behaviour Can Be Effectively Monitored for Change

An Antecedent Behaviour Consequences (the behavioural ABC) chart is an important tool here. It is the foundation of functional analysis and assessment

(Hanley et al., 2003) and enables us to best monitor the implementation and effect of the PBS plan.

In this ABC, the emphasis is based on description of observable events. Here, A is the antecedent or trigger for the challenging or risk behaviour, B is the behaviour or action (the specific observable details about the behaviour) and C is the consequence and response to the behaviour; including a description of how others reacted to the behaviour. This ABC has been integrated into the CBRS-P (Meaden & Hacker, 2010) sheet and now further adapted to enable effective monitoring of PBS plans (see Paul's CBRS-P^{PBS} in Table 7.1). This method of information gathering helps the information to be gathered in a systematic and organised way as clinical notes of past examples are often vague with little indication of potential triggers.

Stage 4: Engaging the Service User and Family

PBS is a collaborative approach. As such it is important to meet with the service user to obtain their perspective and share the emerging plan. Information should be provided about PBS plans as well as highlighting how their behaviour creates a barrier to achieving their goals, thus building motivation for change and collaboration. It is also useful to meet with the family to discuss how sometimes they can inadvertently sabotage intervention efforts, for example by bringing in inappropriate food and drinks. Often, engaging service users in this process may be difficult due to symptoms, cognition or mood. Consequently, multiple attempts may be necessary. However, in the absence of this it may still be helpful to ask others who are involved in the person's care to hypothesise why they believe the behaviour occurs. Carers and family will have access to much useful information about the person often across multiple contexts outside of services and will often need to be engaged if subsequent interventions are to be supported in the community.

Stage 5: Completing the PBS Plan

Once all the relevant information has been gathered, then the team can return and feedback the information they have obtained and try to complete the PBS template (see Table 7.2). The key steps here are:

- Feeding back information from ABC$^{PBS.}$;
- Determining any patterns or trends surrounding when the behaviour occurs. This will help organise staff resources to be able to more readily provide support template (see Table 7.2);
- Agree strategies to put in place when red, amber and green behaviours are present. Strategies should be matched to the function of the behaviour: offering sustained one-to-to time for appropriate behaviours to meet the need for contact. The plan should include three types of proactive strategies:

Table 7.1 Paul's PBS Plan

Red Behaviour: Entering other people's personal space and attempting to or actually touching other people's breasts, bottoms and genital areas

GREEN

What Paul looks like and what he says:

Paul will generally converse with others by asking if they are "alright" repeatedly. He often requires the other person to move the conversation onto other topics and for him to expand on his answers. Paul is *not* repeatedly asking personal questions (e.g. staff's age, where staff live).

Staff support:

1 Staff to recognise and verbally praise Paul when his interactions are appropriate by saying: *"That was a really nice conversation"* or *"It was really nice chatting to you, Paul"*.

AMBER EWS

What Paul looks like and what he says: (early warning signs that Paul may display a "Red" Behaviour)

Paul may ask personal questions (e.g. staff's age, where staff live) or repeatedly comment on others' appearance (e.g. "you look nice today") and/ or use endearing names (e.g. calling staff "babes") while staring, smiling/ laughing and licking his lips. Paul may also become "overfamiliar" (e.g. standing too close, attempting or actually putting an arm around the staff). Paul can minimise this behaviour by stating that he is "only joking".

Staff support:

1 Staff to prompt Paul immediately: *"Paul, please only use my name when greeting me"* or *"That is not an appropriate comment because it makes people uncomfortable"* or *"Paul, you are standing too close to me"* (*demonstrate appropriate/ comfortable distance*).

2 Accept Paul's apology if he provides one.
If Paul states he is only "joking" say: *"All comments are taken seriously and documented and this behaviour cannot continue"*.

3 Staff to engage him in an appropriate topic of conversation (e.g. his plans for the day, movies, books, shopping, his care at the unit, etc.).

4 Praise Paul if he has engaged in an appropriate conversation: *"That was a really nice conversation"* or *"It was really nice chatting to you, Paul"*.

RED

What Paul looks like and what he says:

Paul entering other people's personal space and attempting or actually touching other people's breasts, bottoms and genital area.

Staff support:

1 Staff prompt:
"This behaviour is not okay and you should not touch other's without their permission" or *"Paul, that is not okay. This behaviour will not be tolerated"*.

Table 7.1 (Continued)

BLUE

2 If he states he is only "joking", say:

"*All comments are taken seriously and documented and this behaviour cannot continue*".

3 If Paul does not respond or walks away, allow him some time in a quiet area to ensure that he is calm.

Once Paul is calm

Staff to discuss what happened and what needs to be different to prevent it from happening again (e.g. what are the boundaries, why we have them, meeting his sexual needs in more appropriate ways).

Staff support: Staff to ask:

"*Hi Paul. I hope you are okay? Can we have a chat about what happened earlier on? Can we get a drink?*"

When in quiet space: "*I was informed that you were standing too close to (add person's name)/you touched (person's name) breast today. Can you tell me why that happened?*"

If Paul says he is joking, or "just" or says that he did not touch (person). Staff to say:

"*I understand what you are saying however, you did touch (add name) and they were very upset about it/ or the staff member did not find it funny, in fact they were very upset about it. How does it make you feel when you hear that? Why do you think you feel that way?*"

Staff can say

"*This is a serious offence, as people don't like to be touched in private areas without being asked/people do not like people standing too close to them. Do you understand why they may feel that way? We don't want you to keep getting into trouble, so is there anything you can do to help you avoid this happening in the future?*"

(Offer options/reminders):

1 Go to your room and have some private time?

2 Talk to staff about how you are feeling?

3 Engage in an activity you enjoy? e.g. exercise at the gym?

4 Play PlayStation

5 Go for a walk

Staff can remind Paul where he can get additional support:

"*It may be helpful to talk to the team psychologist if you wish to support you with this behaviour and help you to understand which behaviours are okay and which behaviours are not okay and to see if they can help you to develop more skills to help you when you feel this way?*"

Praise him when he has managed to understand what has been said (positive reinforcement).

Table 7.2 Paul's CBRS-P[PBS]

Red Behaviour (Describe the behaviour as accurately as possible)
Paul grabbed the student nurse's bottom when she was walking up the stairs.

Amber Behaviour (the EWS-R)
What was the service user's presentation and behaviour like leading up to the event in the few hours or minutes before?
Paul was following the student nurse for the past two days. He has been trying to talk to her and said that she looked nice today.

Immediate Trigger
What happened to make the behaviour occur at the particular moment that it did?
Paul was standing in the middle of the stairwell when the student nurse tried to walk past him up the stairs. She asked him to stand to one side, and as she walked past, he grabbed her bottom.

Intervention and Effect? Reactions of Others? (Potential Reinforcers)
What did staff do? What effect did this have?
The student nurse turned and asked Paul why he grabbed at her? Paul just smiled at her and said he was joking and put his hands up in the air.
The student nurse said that "This behaviour is not okay and it's not funny as you should not touch others' without their permission". "I will document this and discuss this with the Nurse in Charge (NIC)".
The student nurse informed the NIC of what happened and the NIC spoke to Paul. The NIC asked why he did what he did. The NIC reinforced that this behaviour is not okay, as it is not okay to touch others without permission.

Service User's View (interview when calm!)
What was [x]'s view of what happened?
Paul said that he touched the student nurse, but "it was a joke".

Blue Strategies Used
NIC met with Paul and said "Hi Paul. I hope you are okay? Can we have a chat about what happened earlier on? Shall we go to a quiet room?"
When in quiet space, "I was informed that you grabbed the student nurses bottom as she was walking up the stairs. Can you tell me why that happened?"
Paul continues to say that he was joking. NIC informed Paul that whilst she understood what Paul was saying, but the student nurse was very upset about it and certainly did not find it funny. He was asked "Why do you think she felt that way?" Paul didn't respond.
NIC also reminded Paul that this is a serious offence, as people don't like to be touched in private areas without being asked and people do not like others following them all day. He was again asked if he understands why she may feel that way. "We don't want you to keep getting into trouble, so is there anything you can do to help you avoid this happening in the future?" "However, if this happens again the police will be informed. We hope that this does not happen. If you feel this way again, can you remember what you can do to avoid getting into trouble?"
Paul was reminded of the other activities he could do:
– Go to your room and have some private time?
– Talk to staff about how you are feeling?
– Engage in activity you enjoy? e.g. exercise at the gym?
– Play PlayStation
– Go for a walk

- *primary or proactive strategies* help to meet the service user's needs and help them learn strategies to communicate their needs effectively;
- *secondary strategies* are designed to prevent escalation to crisis level and to keep the person and others safe. These can include distraction or diversion strategies;
- *tertiary strategies* (reactive strategies) are crisis skills which may include restraints or other restrictive interventions to manage the crisis and reduce the risk of harm to self and others.

A good PBS plan should include more proactive strategies than reactive strategies. Which are used most will depend on the severity of the behaviour expressed.[1] When devising the PBS, it should include a clear definition of the target behaviour titled "Red behaviour" as well as descriptions amber, green and blue behaviours.

- **Green** are primary or proactive strategies that help to meet the service user's needs and to help them learn strategies to communicate their needs effectively;
- **Amber** describes what to do in response to the EWS-R along with guidance on how to intervene;
- **Red** are the operationally defined challenging behaviour that is identified and strategies to manage the behaviour as safely and quickly as possible, to keep the person and those around them safe;
- **Blue** details what to do after the incident occurs and how to help the service user to remain calm and stable.

Once the plan has been created, it should be shared with the whole team, service user and their family. Feedback can then be obtained and any changes made before finalising the plan.

Stage 6: Reviewing the Plan

We regularly review all PBS plans in a reflective practice session space. Here, we review CBRS-P[PBS] sheets to discuss the helpfulness (or unhelpfulness) of the plan with the team. PBS plans are also reviewed in care plan meeting with the service user and their family. In particular it can be helpful to discuss with the team if they believe they have been able to implement the plan. If not, then discussion can be had about what got in the way. If restrictive interventions had to be used, this is an opportunity for the team to reflect on those incidents, explore what happened, develop hypotheses for why this happened and consider what they could do differently next time. If the PBS document needs to be revised, then this can be discussed and planned.

Case Study: Paul

Paul is a 35-year-old male diagnosed with paranoid schizophrenia. He has been under the care of mental health services since the age of 14. Paul has also a mild learning disability. His father died when Paul was young. Shortly afterwards, his mum noticed a change in Paul. He began to express delusional beliefs that the devil was going to hurt him and his family and that he had to protect them. When Paul was 20, he made a suicide attempt by taking an overdose; the devil he said had told him to hurt his family and so he took an overdose in order to kill himself and protect his family. He was taken to a general medical hospital to be treated and then sent to an inpatient acute ward from where after a few weeks he returned back home. By 22, Paul's mental health had deteriorated further and he was sectioned after he disclosed making plans to kill his family to protect them from the devil. He was in psychiatric hospital where he continued to experience voices and was eventually commenced on clozapine. Whilst in hospital, Paul was very unsettled, aggressive and paranoid. He would shout at himself in the mirror, punch and kick walls. He would follow female staff members and would stare at them in ways they found "menacing". He would exhibit sexually inappropriate behaviours by placing his arms across female staff members' chests, stared at female staff and entered their personal space. On one occasion, Paul grabbed a female staff member in her genital area. He also expressed delusional ideas such as believing he was the commander of an army and spoke about believing that it was World War II and that Germany was invading the country. Paul was later transferred to an independent medium secure unit until eventually being transferred to a locked rehabilitation unit. Unfortunately, Paul's clozapine levels would fluctuate due to increased levels of smoking and scoring "red" on his routine blood tests (i.e. white blood cells being much lower than normal, such that patients need to stop taking clozapine immediately). During these periods, Paul's mental health would also fluctuate. It was noted that during such a period, Paul grabbed another female staff member by her genitals. When a new young female staff member joined the team Paul became very interested in her and would follow her around the unit, asking to speak to her. When Paul was getting ready to go out for his escorted leave, he would insist he be taken out by her despite already being allocated another staff member. When asked why he would like this staff member to go with him, he would respond by saying "just".

Other incidences of sexually inappropriate behaviours have included following young male members of staff around the unit and making sexualised comments to them during innocuous conversations. During one such conversation, Paul started to say how attractive he found this staff member and grabbed at his genitals. When asked by the male staff member why he tried to touch him, Paul said that he "was just joking". Paul was reported to be "mentally stable" at the time of these events.

The aforementioned incidences were discussed in reflective practice in the context of completing Paul's START. Staff identified that his sexualised behaviour was the behaviour of most concern. It was frequent, led to restrictions being placed on Paul regarding leave (often leading to Paul becoming angry and abusive) and was little impacted upon by medication. They reported feeling anxious being around him and wanted support on how to manage Paul when he was behaving in this manner. It was agreed that a member from the psychology team together with Paul's named nurse would initially meet with Paul to discuss these recent events.

Paul however repeatedly declined to meet the psychologist. He minimised his behaviour saying that he "didn't do anything" and was "only joking" with the staff members. Paul also expressed some paranoid beliefs towards the psychologist, claiming that they would take his Section 17 leave away from him. It was subsequently agreed that the psychologist would work closely with the named nurse to devise a PBS plan to address Paul's sexualised behaviours. The named nurse could meet with Paul informally and talk through some of the proposed interventions with him.

Devising Paul's PBS Plan

A small team of those most involved in working with Paul was assembled to discuss Paul's behaviour. The Red behaviour was operationalised as:

> Entering other people's personal space and attempting to or actually touching other people's breasts, bottoms and genital areas

The CBRS-P was used to record Paul's behaviour whilst on the unit.

This was then taken back to the whole MDT and Paul himself. Whilst Paul continued to brush off the incidents as jokes, he began to acknowledge that they had happened and that others were actually distressed by them. The consequences for his leave etc. were also explored.

The MDT identified patterns for the triggers for the behaviour. Elements from his START-based CARM formulation were also confirmed. It was agreed that Paul generally had poor social skills and that these had been exacerbated by his time in mental health institutions presenting limited access to appropriate romantic and sexual outlets. His behaviour appeared to be exacerbated by disinhibition associated with a deterioration in mental health.

The team then discussed appropriate strategies, and the named nurse and Paul met to discuss the PBS plan. Once the plan had been revised it was discussed again in reflective practice and at his next care plan meeting. The PBS plan was also documented in Paul's care plan for the whole team to use and for Paul to be aware of what was expected of him.

The CBRS-P^{PBS} sheet was completed to facilitate accurate monitoring of the implementation of the PBS, including relevant PBS elements. The importance of the whole team being familiar with the plan was emphasised alongside the need to accurately document incidents in the CBRS-P^{PBS}.

The PBS plan was reviewed as part of the team's routine three-monthly care plan reviews using the CBRS-P^{PBS} in order to ensure that it was being implemented appropriately. Incidents of the behaviour which were recorded as part of the standard clinical notes system were also reviewed for Paul at these meetings. Over a period of three months, these incidents significantly declined from four to five times per week to only four times during the entire review period.

Summary

In this chapter, we have described how to incorporate PBS into the SAFE approach. The importance of formulating the function of the behaviour and what may be reinforcing this within an MDT approach is critical. Once the behaviour is understood, the PBS process can be used to help the service user learn new ways to meet their needs. PBS is a team-based intervention that requires a consistent committed response from all of those involved. It is perhaps one of the most challenging aspects of implementing SAFE. When effective, it can reduce barriers to recovery as part of a collaborative approach to those with complex mental health and behavioural needs.

It is also a powerful tool to promote the team working together in a compassionate and consistent way to help service users learn new healthy strategies and build better relationships with all members of the MDT.

Note

1 A helpful list of strategies is available on the Challenging Behaviour Foundation website. www.challengingbehaviour.org.uk/

Chapter 8

Using TBCT to Modify the Person's Internal World

Introduction

In Chapter 4, we described how MDTs could utilise information gathered from our various assessment and formulation processes to agree upon relevant care plans aimed at reducing barriers to recovery for our service users. Whilst there is inevitably an overlap, we have come to conceptualise SAFE interventions into two broad categories. TBCT is the first of these and is aimed at those who present with some degree of active engagement or at least prove receptive to team efforts to guide them away from engaging in problem behaviours and questioning their motives (e.g. challenging the perceived need to comply with command hallucinations). The second category concerns a broader range of interventions, partly behavioural, partly social, involving primarily team efforts to intervene with setting events, triggers and reinforcers. We term these "internal" and "external" interventions that are focused on internal (mental) and external events drawn from our CARM formulation. Ideally, internal interventions can be offered, as these arguably have greater potential for promoting lasting and more generalisable change. However, external interventions acknowledge that our service users are part of a wider social system (e.g. family, rehabilitation team members) and that systemic change can also have meaningful and significant impacts for them.

Key Features of TBCT

The initial work on TBCT (Meaden & Hacker, 2010) focused primarily on what we now term active behaviours. We have since attempted to use SAFE to address behaviours more closely associated with negative symptoms (Fox & Meaden, 2015) or passive behaviours, utilising TBCT approaches. In this chapter, we outline our evolving understanding of working with active and passive behaviours using internal interventions, such as TBCT.

Despite ongoing research efforts and anecdotal evidence to the contrary, there remains a lack of robust evidence to make firm conclusions regarding the effectiveness of adding CBT to standard care for people with schizophrenia compared to standard care alone (Jones et al., 2018). However, the ABC cognitive therapy

DOI: 10.4324/9781003082811-9

model of psychosis continues to garner evidence that strongly supports the relationship between voice-related beliefs and harmful behaviour (Birchwood et al., 2017). Problems with generalisability to routine clinical settings persist, especially for hard-to-reach populations. We offer TBCT as one alternative to address some of these problems. We propose that there are several benefits of adopting this more team-based form of cognitive therapy.

1   It serves to increase the amount of CBT-P offered from what is usually once a week at best to potentially daily or even several times each day.
2   It targets distress and problem behaviour beliefs that are most active (in-situation beliefs) which we have proposed are the immediate drivers of distress and problem behaviour.
3   MDT staff become co-therapists, socialising them into the cognitive model, increasing their understanding of the individual's problems and what drives them and utilises established alliances between individuals and those most engaged with them.
4   It targets beliefs held by team members who interfere with care.

The core components of TBCT can be summarised as:

1   Adoption of the cognitive ABC formulation to form the underlying core model. Here, **A** is the **a**ctivating event, **B** the **b**eliefs or appraisals for these events and **C** the emotional and behavioural **c**onsequences of these beliefs (Chadwick et al., 1996)
2   "Pan-situational beliefs"

These are stable beliefs present across a range of situations. In CBT-P they effectively constitute stable dynamic factors, but in TBCT we conceptualise them more as static factors. They include beliefs about the person, others and the world (including psychotic beliefs). Pan-situational beliefs tend to be static, functioning as vulnerability factors which give rise to specific interpretations in specific situations. They do not necessarily lead directly to distress and problem behaviours;

3   "In-situation beliefs"

In our model, these are the immediate drivers of distress and behaviour and function as acute dynamic risk factors. They constitute inferences about what is happening and may include so-called cognitive biases such as jumping to conclusions (e.g. Moritz & Woodward, 2005). These are the key targets of TBCT, linking most clearly to EWS-R and as such, afford the opportunity to modify reactions to both external and internal setting events

4   Disputation (the **D** in our cognitive therapy model) is best delivered in the situations in which distress and behaviour are present

5   Interlinking the team's beliefs and behaviour with that of the individual. Here, the individual's behaviours are the activating events (the A in our model) for the team's beliefs about them and their behaviour (its assumed function), for example *"they are doing this to gain attention because they are manipulative"* (see Chapter 6, Figure 6.3)

6   The team's beliefs are legitimate targets for intervention since they lead to unhelpful care responses or behaviours which mitigate against delivering consistent effective and recovery-focused interventions

7   Care plans in our TBCT model become the Experiment or **E**, testing out the new understanding of the function of each behaviour

8   Formulation (the **F** in our cognitive therapy model) serves not only to guide intervention plans but also to **D**ispute unhelpful team beliefs where appropriate. This is a careful and sensitive process building on the SAFE clinicians' relationship with the team which needs to be established over time.

Case Illustration: Atif

Atif frequently hears voices telling him to hit others who they tell him are going to attack him today (the **A**ctivating event). The team members believed that Atif primarily hits others when he is in a bad mood. When other residents are gathered in large numbers (a key setting event), it triggers his belief that an attack is imminent and the in-situation **B**elief: "I must do what my voice says otherwise I will be hurt". Atif begins walking with his back to the walls and clenching his fists (the Behavioural **C**onsequence; a threat mitigation safety behaviour). The staff alert to these EWS-R and then intervene by asking Atif if the voices are warning him again. They encourage him to remember that he has actually never been attacked by them even when he is "not on his guard" and that the voices are unreliable (TBCT – **D**isputation). Atif trusts some members of the staff who are chosen for delivering this intervention. Atif is not attacked and does not hit anyone. This provides further evidence that the voices get things wrong. It also demonstrates to the staff that it is the voices that drive this behaviour, not just being in a bad mood (the **E**xperiment outcome).

9   **G** is the care plan Goal

10   Finally, **H** emphasises the importance of holding **H**ope.

Aims, Stages and Techniques for Active Behaviours

Aims

Our initial aim is to align the individual's and staff's ABC, thus relocating the problem to the individual's A-B rather than the team's C-B explanation (their functional explanation of the individual's distress and behaviour). Secondly, we aim to shift the focus away from any negative responses to the problem behaviour to interventions that address the true function of the problem behaviour.

Understanding the function of the behaviour enables the team to address each of the factors which drives it. TBCT primarily targets internal setting events and internal triggers: the individual's in-situation appraisals of what is happening or likely to happen and the need to deal with it in a particular way.

Stages

In keeping with our theme of parallel processes, we outline the key stages for both individuals and teams for developing a shared TBCT-based care plan.

1   The assessment and initial formulation process place the **C** at the beginning. This emphasises the notion that it is distress and behaviour that are the targets and not symptoms (which are actually **As** in our cognitive model). Each problem behaviour potentially has its own specific in-situation belief/s. Clarifying the behaviour as the starting point is important if the intervention is to be accurately targeted.

2   The **CAB** framework can be used to elicit both immediate and distant triggers, but this requires separating out the As further. When discussing concerns with the person it is often helpful to agree to a specific event to examine, one in which the person was experiencing distress and/or engaged in a behaviour which everyone (including ideally the person) agreed was problematic. Where engagement does not allow a discussion with the individual, the SAFE practitioner and the team must hypothesise (often based on anecdotes derived from interactions with the individual) what the in-situation beliefs are and tentatively try to clarify with the person when EWS-R are present what they might be: "*Are you okay Atif? You seem a bit on edge. Are the voices bothering you?*"

3   Disputing the service user's hypothetical Bs as part of the team's subsequent TBCT efforts will need to be even more sensitively approached. Some time may need to be taken at this stage in arriving at a consensus regarding which behaviour is most usefully targeted. Individuals and different team members will likely have differing views on this. It is helpful to consider which behaviour might be most amenable to change, which is most frequent (providing the opportunity to intervene), which creates the most barriers to recovery for the individual (see also Chapter 7).

4   Where a sufficient degree of engagement allows, we attempt to elicit the actual **A** from the individual's perspective. This clarifies whether or not the behaviour is being driven by objectively understandable setting events and triggers or whether the behaviour is being driven by psychotic interpretations of innocuous events (aligned with pan-situational static/vulnerability beliefs). Care team members often struggle to understand behaviour that is not clearly driven by obvious external events. It is vital therefore to understand the

individual's internal world and how this interacts with the external world as shared by others.

5   Next, we attempt to elicit the individual's **B-C** explanation (belief and behaviour) and the **Ce** (the emotional consequence). By continuing to focus on a particular event when the person was distressed or engaged in the behaviour, we can ask a number of leading questions:

What was it about the event that upset you/seemed to upset them so much?
What did you think was happening?
What was it about the situation that meant you/them behaved in this particular way?

We may subsequently try to identify and examine similar incidents over a relevant recent period in order to clarify if the in-situation belief is part of a consistent pattern.

6.   Next, we attempt to uncover the actual **A** which led to the interpretation or belief. When trying to establish **the A-B** link, clarifying questions are often helpful:

"*So A happened and you took that to mean B?*"

We may then reflect back the information from this process as an **A-B-C chain**: "*So A happened, and you took that to mean B, and you felt/did C?*"

This step begins the process of socialising the person into the model making them more receptive to TBCT.

7   The next stage is to elicit the team's ABC which begins the process of disputing team member's beliefs. Potentially, carers too can be involved in this process. We turn again to the agreed target behaviour and distress (**Ce** and **Cb**). Team members are encouraged to express their own views about the causes or reasons for a given individual's behaviour (team members **A-B**) without prejudice or disputation. Rather it is emphasised that all views are valued.

8   TBCT is primarily centred around our CARM models (Meaden et al., 2015; Fox & Meaden, 2015). Our CARM model for active behaviours first developed by Meaden and Hacker (2010) provides multiple points of intervention where social/environmental cognitive and behavioural factors interact. TBCT essentially targets internal factors. Whilst we have anchored this primarily to early warning signs, potentially TBCT could be offered at different points.

Internal Setting Events

Supporting the service user to reappraise their in-situation beliefs in the presence of EWS-R; for example Baily believes that a specific member of staff in the garden area of the unit is watching her with the intent of harming her.

Internal Triggers

Supporting the service user to address more acute threat-related beliefs; for example Baily feels a pain in her chest (the TBCT target) which is an anxiety symptom. Baily however believes that this is the member of staff attacking her with radiation. She assaults them believing that this is the best way to stop the attack.

Internal Reinforcers

Baily feels calmer believing that she has thwarted the attack. However, this serves as a safety behaviour (the TBCT target) preventing her from learning that the attack is not real but rather is a symptom of anxiety. Baily's belief that violence can be an acceptable interpersonal solution is both an in-situation belief and also a belief developed in childhood (a vulnerability factor). This is another TBCT target which also affords the opportunity to tackle a more deep-seated antisocial belief.

TBCT Techniques

In order to enlist team members as co-therapists, the formulation process will need to effectively dispute any unhelpful team beliefs about the service user and their behaviour. The sharing and live devising of the service user's possible ABCs aim to socialise the team into the cognitive model and show its power as an explanatory framework. Subsequently, a number of techniques can be useful in eliciting team ABCs and enlisting them as co-therapists:

1   *Systemic techniques* from family therapy involving circular questioning can be helpful here, encouraging team members to reflect on their beliefs in the light of the emerging formulation. Circular questioning is used to "*invite participants into a conversation to consider relational aspects of the topic being investigated*" (Evans & Whitcombe, 2015, p. 28) and help them see alternatives, other options and possibilities and explore other people's views. Unlike "linear questions" (our "What. . .?" questions) which aim to elicit facts and content and determine information about the situation, circular questioning encourages reflection and exploration. Evans and Whitcombe (2015) describe several types of useful circular questions. Two of these we have found particularly useful.

Temporal Questions

These encourage reflection on what has happened in the past, any changes that have taken place over time along with the details regarding an event. They also involve exploration of optimism or pessimism and invite consideration of a time in the future when things might be different or improved.

Triadic Questions

These invite reflection regarding how two people's actions impact upon the behaviour or mood of another.

2   **Dividing up tasks** aids the process of clarifying and agreeing the various components of the CARM formulation template and also instils curiosity and the suspension of beliefs about the person and their behaviour. The strategy here is to realign team ABCs to the individual's ABC. This involves:

    a   Gathering information from all known case notes;
    b   Direct observation;
    c   Informal interviews during the course of other activities, asking gentle enquiring questions regarding any worries or problems the person may be experiencing;
    d   Formal interviews: post incident review with the person and others involved.

This process aims to provide evidence to confirm or disconfirm hypotheses regarding the functions of the behaviour and reveal more pertinent intervention targets. Where consensus cannot be reached regarding formulation elements, the SAFE clinician should adopt a pragmatic stance acknowledging that not all competing theories can be resolved at this stage. The effectiveness of interventions may help to resolve existing uncertainties: any subsequent change in the individual's behaviour provides evidence that the new understanding has some validity, thus acting as an Experiment (**E**) and further Disputing (**D**) the team's beliefs.

3   **Team members are taught basic techniques** for eliciting beliefs and empathising with the individual's emotional responses using reflection, paraphrasing and suspension of disbelief. They are then taught how to identify the actual A when they observe any EWS-R. Typical questions may include:

    a   "What did [x] do to indicate that they were doing this (e.g., persecuting you)?"
    b   "How did you figure this out?" (Avoiding words like "think" or "believe", which discredit the individual's experience).

This enables team members to clarify the actual **A** and feed this back as an **ABC**: the real event (**A**), the individual's interpretation of it (**B**) and their resulting feelings and behaviour (**Ce** and **Cb**). Subsequent possible alternative explanations or interpretations of the **A** can then be elicited or suggested. This reinterpretation of **A** utilises traditional cognitive therapy procedures:

a   Eliciting supporting evidence and weighing it – fairly examining the evidence
b   Examining alternatives

c   Exploring logical inconsistencies
d   Testing out beliefs.

These stages, strategies and techniques are illuminated through the case study of Steve.

Case Study: Steve

To illustrate the process of TBCT we return to our case study Steve, first introduced in Chapter 5. Here, our focus is on illustrating the TBCT process. Steve being violent towards others – punching or hitting others – remains the target behaviour. However, to prevent future occurrences, it was agreed to focus on incidents of verbal abuse and threats to harm, since these tended to constitute EWS-R for actual physical violence. A particular recent incident around mealtime was examined, as this is a setting which had previously escalated to physical assault; mealtimes were a common trigger-point for Steve.

Eliciting the ABCs

Steve's named nurse sat down with him and asked what was it about this event that made him so angry and threatens to hurt staff members. Steve said that he believes staff were against him, laughing at him and wanted to control him. With gentle non-judgemental encouragement the nurse was able to clarify the ABC with Steve (see Table 8.1).

Table 8.1 Steve's ABC

Activation event	**B**eliefs *(In-situation)*	**C**onsequences *(emotional and behavioural*
At mealtime, Steve is refused a second helping of food. *(There were no extra portions available that day.)*	Staff are deliberately denying me food, they planned this to upset me and laugh at me *(In-situation belief)*. ⬆ Others want to control me. Others don't care about me. *(Paranoid Vulnerability Belief)*	Gets angry at staff, swears at them and threatens to hit them. Staff intervene and sometimes restrain him.

In a reflective practice session, the same exercise was carried out, with staff focusing on the same incident. Staff were invited so explain how (the behavioural C) and why (their Beliefs) they had responded as they had and how they felt. Emphasising the staff's emotional reactions helps to build motivation in the staff team by working towards reducing their distress.

The TBCT

Using circular questioning techniques, the team reflected on their beliefs in light of the formulation. This process aims to confirm and disconfirm hypotheses regarding the function of the behaviour. At this point, the SAFE clinician was able to refer back to Steve's narrative CARM formulation (see Chapter 5) and review the recent mealtime incident in light of this. Explicitly drawing out these comparisons is important, as having previously formulated this behaviour does not necessarily lead to change in the assumptions held by team members. This can be for a number of reasons:

1   The START process and subsequent SAFE formulations cover a range of behaviours and involve multiple levels of process and so such insights are often lost in the bigger picture
2   In the heat of the moment, staff members may revert to viewing such situations in terms of their own pan-situational beliefs and will tend to reason emotionally when threatened in this way. This can then lead to biases such as jumping to conclusions.

Setting events were then reviewed. For Steve, these would typically involve getting up late (having missed breakfast) and there being minimal snacks available. Note that the EWS-R for this behaviour will differ slightly from the actual target behaviour of physical violence. They will in effect be the EWS-R for the EWS-P.

Table 8.2 Steve's Staff's ABC

Activating event	Beliefs (attributional biases)	Consequences (emotional and behavioural)
Steve gets angry at the staff, swears at them and threatens to push or hit them	He provokes others deliberately because he is just looking for a fight and to get attention. He is not hungry and will sell or trade the food items. He is diabetic and needs to lose weight.	Staff feel intimidated and annoyed. Some staff walk away, and others challenge him, telling him that he can't have seconds as he is overweight and needs to go on a diet. *Reinforces Steve's beliefs that the staff want to control him and they don't care about him.*

Steve can moreover appear irritable in mood (exacerbated by hunger) with a hostile facial expression.

Agreeing Co-therapist TBCT Techniques

TBCT techniques, whilst primarily aimed at addressing in-situation beliefs linked to setting events, can be further refined. We illustrate TBCT techniques employed at different stages of the behaviour in Steve's TBCT plan (see Table 8.3):

A more detailed set of questions and cognitive challenges was also devised, especially for the staff when conducting a post incident review with Steve.

*   When you say that the staff want to get you into trouble, what indicated this to you?
*   How did you figure this out?
*   What would be the problem if things were to continue as they are?
*   Could there be another explanation for why the staff did not give you a second helping of food?

Table 8.3 Steve's ABC TBCT Plan

Activating (setting events and triggers)	**B**elief (realigned to Steve's actual insinuation B)	**C**onsequences (emotional and behavioural)
Steve arrives late for lunch having overslept and missed breakfast. He complains of being hungry, is agitated and has an angry facial expression. Steve asks for an extra portion, but it is not available and is angry, abusive and threatening when he is not given one.	He thinks we are against him. Didactic dispute: "*It's nothing personal Steve*". Calmly explain to him and show him that there are no extra portions today. Encourage him to have something healthy instead: a piece of fruit.	Show understanding and compassion. The staff offer bowl of fruit to choose a piece. The staff sit with Steve afterwards (when he is calm) to explain and ask if there is anything they can do to help him to meet his goals of staying calm when refused such requests.
Early Intervention *The staff to approach Steve before he gets to the canteen hatch and ask if he is okay, acknowledge he may be hungry and explain that there may not be any extra food today but remind him that there is always extra fruit afterwards.*		

- What could the staff say to you to show that they are concerned for you that you would be open to listening to?
- What could the staff say or do when you miss breakfast and wake up late and you are feeling hungry and want more food?
- What would be the best way to move forward so that you and the staff do not get upset around mealtimes?

Other Supporting Interventions

The named nurse met with Steve to understand more about his poor sleep. Steve said that even though he goes to bed at around 10 p.m., he does not actually sleep until 2 a.m. He said that he drinks coffee and watches a movie or plays on his PlayStation until late. The named nurse asked if Steve wanted to wake up on time for breakfasts to which he said he did. It was also highlighted that with diabetes, Steve needed to eat regularly. They agreed to look at changing his sleep pattern so that he was not sleeping too late and was able to wake up on time for breakfast. This included no caffeinated tea, coffee or energy drinks after 6 p.m., but it was agreed that he could have decaffeinated coffee. Steve started some sleep hygiene work with the occupational therapist, with whom he also got on well.

TBCT for Passive Behaviours

What we now term passive behaviours have traditionally been most closely associated with the so-called negative symptoms of schizophrenia. These can be summarised briefly as blunted affect, poverty of speech, social withdrawal, avolition and anhedonia (Andreasen, 1982). CBT-P efforts have predominantly focused on managing the impact of delusions and voices which are generally linked with active problem behaviours such as violence and self-harm. However, whilst having some impact on risk behaviours (e.g. Birchwood et al., 2014) CBT-P benefits have not been translated into improved long-term functional outcomes (Robinson et al., 2004). A failure to engage in activities of daily living, work and education is in part attributable to negative symptoms (Wykes & Reeder, 2006). There is a need to better target psychological interventions towards the specific mechanisms and beliefs linked to passive behaviours. In some cases, passive behaviours may actually be related to the so-called positive symptoms of psychosis, also referred to as "secondary negative symptoms" (Kirschner et al., 2017).

Case Illustration: Gary

Gary's voices tell him to not to talk to others or show his feelings as they will steal his words and his mind. He speaks little and merely mumbles when spoken to (poverty of speech) and avoids social interaction (social withdrawal).

Case Illustration: Kerry

Kerry has delusional beliefs that secret agents will kidnap her while she is asleep at night. She therefore pretends to sleep but actually stays awake most of the night. During the day, Kerry presents as lethargic, lacking any interest in engaging in activities (avolition and anhedonia).

These mediating beliefs can be targeted using TBCT once they are identified. They are less amenable to early warning signs planning since they tend to be continuous behaviours, lacking obvious setting events and triggers. Carefully eliciting and understanding Gary and Kerry's internal worlds is essential here. Such intervention is possible only through the patient and careful building of a therapeutic relationship.

In developing TBCT for passive behaviours not linked to specific delusions or voices, we have drawn upon developments in the psychological understanding of negative symptoms, which have been introduced in Chapter 6 with the CARM formulation for passive behaviours. Foussias and Remington (2010) proposed a key role for avolition (an inability to initiate and maintain goal-directed behaviour). They argue that the different domains through which negative symptoms can be experienced are fundamentally linked to a reduction in the appetitive drive (or "wanting"). Without this drive, individuals are said to no longer be motivated to engage in goal-directed behaviour, even though the consummatory drive (i.e. "liking") remains intact. In other words, individuals can still enjoy activities but do not appear to want to engage in them. Understanding this paradigm shift further, we turned to the work exploring dysfunctional thinking biases regarding performance expectancy in people with psychosis (Fox & Meaden, 2015).

Beck and colleagues have outlined a theoretical framework for negative symptoms structured around negative beliefs about the self and others. They argue that primary negative symptoms are an extreme version of premorbid personality patterns – particularly schizoid and schizotypal traits (Beck & Rector, 2005; Rector et al., 2005). Such primary negative symptoms can arise independently of positive symptoms of psychosis and often reflect generally low expectations of pleasure, achievement and acceptance by others (Beck & Rector, 2005). Rector et al. (2005) outline four types of cognitive expectancy:

1   Low expectancies for pleasure
2   Low expectancies for success
3   Low expectancies for acceptance
4   A perception of limited resources.

These expectancies interact, such as the belief that one has low ability in an area (perception of limited resource) reduces the expectation of success and that others will accept you. As negative symptoms worsen, negative expectancy appraisals are reinforced.

A developing evidence base has emerged supporting the targeting of CBT interventions towards these appraisals (see Elis et al., 2013 for a review). However, it is also important to consider the role of reduced cognitive resources in the maintenance of negative symptoms, particularly the role of cognitive deficits in schizophrenia.

Cognitive Deficits

There is now a large body of literature that suggests problems in processing information in people with psychosis (e.g. Bora et al., 2010). Despite considerable heterogeneity in the types of cognitive deficits described (Palmer et al., 2009), it is now acknowledged that these are important targets for intervention (Pfammatter et al., 2011). In their meta-analysis of studies, Fett, et al. (2011) identified a range of cognitive domains associated with poor functional outcomes:

- Neuro-cognitive deficits (e.g. learning, memory and processing speed);
- Social-cognitive deficits (e.g. theory of mind, social perception), with theory of mind deficits being the most strongly associated with poorer community functioning.

Reduced abilities to process information would not only serve to provide fertile ground for reinforcing negative outcome expectancies (e.g. through failed tasks due to limited cognitive resources), but they could also reduce the chances of people being able to effectively engage in cognitive behavioural therapeutic work (e.g. cognitive reasoning, or carrying out homework tasks, where social cognitive deficits would impair functional performance). In order to most appropriately design interventions towards those with negative symptoms and passive behaviours, three key areas emerge:

1 Low self-efficacy beliefs
2 Negative outcome expectancies
3 Remediation of cognitive difficulties.

Both cognitive remediation (Wykes et al., 2011) and social-cognitive training therapies (Kurtz & Richardson, 2012) have shown some promise here. However, in isolation these interventions appear to have limited effects on broader functional outcomes showing quite specific effects on premorbid IQ, baseline cognition and training task progress (Reser et al., 2019). This suggests that further intervention is required to maximise and broaden potential benefits. Consequently, these form an ideal candidate for TBCT. Our aims are to translate these research findings into everyday practice for those who are simply not receptive to traditionally delivered psychosocial approaches. TBCT uses the CARM formulation to harness the resources of the team and has the potential to offer frequent intervention in everyday life situations.

Passive behaviours relate closely to Beck's proposal of primary negative symptom. TBCT can be usefully applied to support other formulation-driven team interventions to maximise functional outcomes. We outline our revised TBCT framework later and show how the emerging evidence-based strategies can be integrated into an effective treatment approach for those who are hard to reach and treat.

Aims, Stages and Techniques for Passive Behaviours

When formulating passive behaviours which tend to be continuous the ability to identify and target early warning signs is not feasible or is arguably less relevant. Instead, our focus has been on the role of internal mental events that maintain the experience of avolition (or lack of goal-directed behaviour). Rector et al. (2005) appear to position expectancy beliefs as more enduring and therefore stable personality-based beliefs. In our CARM model these would now constitute vulnerability factors, and as with delusional beliefs we suggest that they give rise to or create the conditions for specific in-situation beliefs. The theory of Rector et al. (2005) supports at least four broad types of in-situation beliefs relevant to the maintenance of passive behaviours.

1   Low Expectancies for Pleasure

Rector et al. (2005) provide evidence that people with psychosis report lower appetitive pleasure but similar consummatory pleasure compared to a control group (see also Gard et al., 2007). Consequently, individuals with psychosis have minimal motivation for pleasurable activities as they do not expect to enjoy them.

2   Low Expectancies for Success

Cognitive deficits associated with psychosis may make failure at tasks more likely, so it is important to understand the standards that individuals are attempting to meet. Rector et al. (2005) also highlight how individuals may be judging their performance in meeting their own expectations as well as those of other people. Cognitive factors such as hypervigilance to criticism and memory biases can serve to maintain these beliefs.

3   Low Acceptance

The stigma of a diagnosis of schizophrenia can be profound, with many individuals reporting feelings of shame (Knight et al., 2003, p. 214). This may fuel negative self-evaluative beliefs with individuals viewing themselves as inferior to others and there being little point in trying to overcome challenges. These pan-situational beliefs are likely to further underpin reduced expectancies for success which in turn behaviourally results in avoidance for fear of being judged negatively (Rector et al., 2005).

4   Perception of Limited Resources

As Rector et al. (2005) point out, beliefs about having diminished resources in cognitive, social and material domains tend to be exaggerated and inflexible. In conjunction with low expectations of success and negative appraisal by others, behavioural avoidance of activities may become firmly established safety behaviours, limiting distress in the short term but preventing exposure to disconfirmatory experiences.

Aims

Expectancy beliefs are pan-situational evaluative beliefs about the self, others and the world. Accompanying behaviours tend to be largely continuous. However, as with delusional beliefs they are not acted on all of the time and in all situations; if they did, the person would simply not function at all and would require high levels of continuing nursing care. Incorporating these beliefs into a modified CARM model (Fox & Meaden, 2015), we find that it is the specific nature of the task faced and the individual's in-situation beliefs about the particular task that determine their behavioural response. Addressing these is our aim in TBCT for passive behaviours. Longer-term individual therapy may become possible in order to address evaluative pan-situational beliefs, often after several formulations of different behaviours have gathered evidence that can be used to create cognitive dissonance in individual CBT-P sessions. Successful application of TBCT may usefully provide evidence that contradicts the core expectancy beliefs. It is also important to note that other (non-cognitive) internal and external factors may contribute to the expression and maintenance of passive behaviours. These external barriers can be identified in our SLF. These may limit the opportunity to address in-situation expectancies such that the person is prevented from gaining access to situations and activities that may challenge them; for example limited opportunity to mix with others of an appropriate cultural or religious disposition due to lack of staffing to facilitate community leave or being placed in a setting remote from such opportunities.

Stages

1   The initial task is to identify which tasks and activities or situations the person anticipates being judged negatively in and which expectancies are pertinent: expectancy of low acceptance and/or low expectancy of success.
2   We can then proceed to identify which activities, tasks or situations the person associates with expectancies of success, pleasure and/or acceptance.
3   Different expectations may be pertinent to different passive behaviours. Consequently, as with active behaviours, the team will need to be clear

about which passive behaviour they are going to formulate and target for intervention.

4   It is important therefore to consider several different examples of passive behaviours in order to be able to formulate the different outcome expectancies. Behavioural observations are the main method here. The skills of occupational therapists are particularly helpful in terms of assessing the functional skills and deficits of individuals with passive behaviours, especially as they relate to activities of daily living.

9   Utilising the CAB framework to elicit both immediate and distant triggers.

10   Identifying the individual's cognitive ABC by examining a specific example of not engaging in or performing an activity. With passive behaviours, emotional consequences may be less readily apparent but are usually there such as hopelessness, shame or despair.

11   Identifying and examining similar incidents over a relevant recent period in order to clarify if the in-situation belief is part of a consistent pattern.

12   Eliciting the team's cognitive ABC is the next stage, sensitively eliciting with compassionate curiosity team member's views about the causes or reasons for the individual's behaviour (team members A-B) without challenging them directly.

13   As with active behaviours, some information gathering will likely be required to examine the evidence to support and test different hypotheses.

14   Planning the intervention is the final stage. Here, the individual's in-situation beliefs (hypothesised or directly elicited) are targeted whenever the behaviour is present or an activity is agreed, planned and encouraged.

Techniques

Once the relevant expectancies have been identified and formulated, work can begin on devising TBCT strategies. In-situation expectancy beliefs are in effect predictions or inferences. Consequently, the same CBT-P techniques that are applied to addressing inferences can be applied here:

1   Eliciting supporting evidence and weighing it – fairly examining the evidence
2   Examining alternatives
3   Exploring logical inconsistencies
4   Testing out beliefs.

Importantly, because the consummatory drive (liking) is intact (Foussias & Remington, 2010), behavioural experiments or behavioural activation can be designed and planned that works on the intrinsic reward of pleasurable activities. Taking part in meaningful activities in a safe, non-judgemental environment can be used as both a self-reinforcing pleasurable intervention and also as an opportunity to test out negative expectations. An important caveat here is to acknowledge that some of these inferences expressed by the service user may indeed be accurate – such as the experience of stigma. These need to be acknowledged and validated. Ultimately, the goal here is to help the individual inoculate themselves against these. Work on self-evaluative thinking, if possible, may usefully involve learning to down rank and reduce the power of others' inferences and evaluations. Often, people affected by psychosis will see themselves in a subordinate position to others and consequently, others are perceived as having more power (Meaden et al., 2012) and their views of the person seem more persuasive and true. As such, techniques from cognitive therapy for command hallucinations may be helpful here (Meaden et al., 2012):

1   Down ranking the other:

> *"Just because X (the powerful other) said this or made you feel this way it does not automatically make it true or true forever"*.
> *"They are fallible human beings just like anyone else"*.
> *"Perhaps they have faults of their own?"*

2   Labels are not facts:

> Here, analogies can be helpful. The person can be encouraged to think about the general issues of labelling things and how this can be wrong or misleading at times: buying fake designer sunglasses from the market.

3   Examining the intent of the powerful other:

> Thinking about others' reasons for holding such prejudicial beliefs can help the person to consider that others' points of view may belie hurtful or malicious intentions rather than being a statement of fact. In which case why take any notice of them. Or perhaps they are just simply ignorant!

We illustrate these stages and techniques in the following case study.

Case Study: Luke

Luke is a 45-year-old Black British male who is soon to be discharged into the community from a long-term placement in a HDU. Luke was admitted into services after concerned neighbours called an ambulance when he became locked out of his flat, appearing unwashed and dishevelled, with jumbled speech and disorganised thought content. Luke lived alone, with no friends in the local community; his family lived overseas in the Caribbean. In services, Luke presented as suspicious and wary, becoming verbally and physically aggressive on some occasions (primarily towards staff and other service users). This appeared to be driven by persecutory paranoia and expectations that others would take advantage of him. These positive symptoms of psychosis appeared to dissipate following stabilisation on a suitable medication regime. There has been little evidence of paranoia and no incidents of aggression in the last six months. Luke has required active support from the staff to attend to his daily hygiene needs (e.g. shower, brush teeth, change his clothes) and also has a tendency to store food inappropriately (e.g. buying raw chicken and storing this in his bedroom cupboard). These needs have responded somewhat to skills training and active monitoring from the staff, such that Luke is preparing to move into a supported living placement in his own flat. This placement was agreed with Luke due to it being in an area he is familiar and happy with; however, the support available on site is not 24 hours. Luke's new AOT are concerned that he will be vulnerable in the community as he has no family in the country and has no way of contacting the team if he needs to. Luke does not use a mobile phone and reports never having used one. Luke has dismissed the idea of having a mobile phone as it is "too expensive" and "too complicated".

Stages

In the development of the TBCT plan, a small case formulation team was assembled comprising inpatient staff who have worked closely with Luke, alongside Luke's care coordinator and the occupational therapist from the AOT. It was agreed that the main target would be the use of the mobile phone as this could be a key useful resource for Luke to access support and maintain his safety in the community.

The initial hypothesis was that Luke's decision to not use a mobile phone may be partly due to expectancy of lack of success with this (i.e. "too complicated"). It also appeared that Luke was unaware that he could potentially use his phone to access video clips that he enjoys (he enjoyed martial arts films). It was noted that Luke does seem to experience some cognitive deficits, such as slow processing speed and poor recall of new information. It was hypothesised that these may also maintain the avoidance of learning new skills due to perceived slow progress and lack of success (e.g. Luke continues to struggle to learn new recipes during his cooking sessions at the unit). External factors were quickly identified as the pressure to get Luke discharged into the community and the anxiety staff felt about his discharge. A team-focussed cognitive ABC identified that this anxiety was linked to beliefs about Luke's inability to manage in the community and the implications of relapse:

A: Discharge planning for Luke (inference: we must get this right);
B: Luke can't cope; if he relapses, all this work will be lost; it is safer for Luke in a residential placement;
C: Anxiety, worry, delay discharge.

In a one-to-one session, the psychologist and care coordinator discussed with Luke his views about the use of the mobile phone. Luke explained that he did not need a phone to contact people as there was "no-one to speak to" and the process of using a phone was "too complicated" and he would not be able to "get my head around it". Luke also saw little point in using a phone as he had "no-one" to talk to. It became clear that Luke was unaware of the ability to use the phone to do various other activities, such as watch video clips, nor that calling family members overseas was readily accessible using free Wi-Fi-based apps. Luke speaks with his mother in Jamaica every fortnight, when she rings him on the unit phone in the evening. Luke expressed interest in the idea of a video call with his mother when this was suggested, as he had not seen her for many years. A CARM formulation was developed (see Figure 8.1).

The staff team reflected on how their beliefs and worries mirrored some of Luke's own negative expectations of himself (that he cannot cope/use a mobile phone) and noted that one of the consequences was a focus on restrictive placements, which although "safe", limited Luke's freedom and opportunity. It was also noted that while some of these concerns were based on evidence (e.g. Luke did experience cognitive difficulties that impacted his speed in learning new skills), the team's response was overly restrictive and limited the options for Luke, who wanted to leave hospital. It was agreed that using a mobile phone would be one good way of being able to access support and resources in the community. As a first step, Luke agreed to use a unit computer to try to speak to his mother in Jamaica over a video connection and reported that he enjoyed seeing her. Importantly, Luke's mother was also very pleased to see Luke, and they arranged future monthly video chats with her and his brother, who lived close to his mother in Jamaica.

One-to-one sessions were spent working with Luke to explain the options that a mobile phone offers, including video calls and watching video clips. Luke agreed that he enjoyed seeing his mother, and the possibility of continuing this contact on discharge (in the new accommodation) was discussed. Luke expressed concern about ever being able to know how to use a smartphone that allows video calls, particularly his ability to remember all the functions and buttons on the phone. With support from the AOT occupational therapist, a bespoke manual was developed to guide Luke in using a simple smartphone that included photos of the phone and a step-by-step guide for each function. Weekly sessions were used for Luke to practise with staff using the phone and the manual. Initially, these

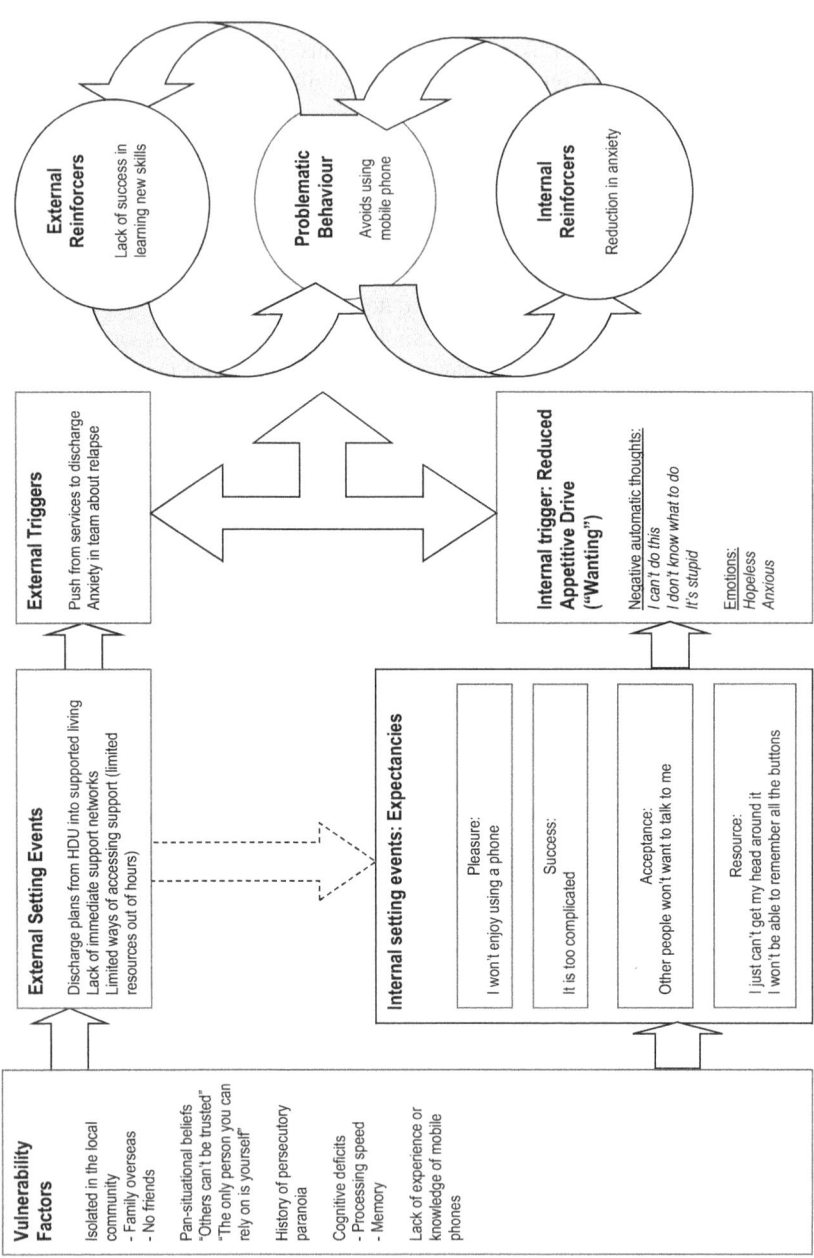

Figure 8.1 CARM Formulation of Luke Not Using a Mobile Phone

sessions were weekly and went through the different steps required for the functions Luke wanted to use upon discharge: making phone calls, video calls, texting family and watching video clips.

Luke quickly found that he enjoyed watching martial arts clips on the video player and was motivated to learn which local shops and cafes had free Wi-Fi so as not to incur charges when he was out. It was noticed that Luke liked to follow the same steps of the same skills in sessions, and the ability to make calls and watch videos had a self-reinforcing function, with Luke expressing his pleasure at completing the steps. Attention was drawn to Luke's ability to use the phone and the pleasure associated with this (i.e. gently highlighting the mismatch between expectation and outcome). Using the manual, weekly sessions were increased to three times a week to increase the "dosage" of skills training to help improve both skill and confidence, ready for discharge. It was noted that Luke was always on time for his "phone sessions", and that for the staff, it was one of the "highlights of the week". Exploration of this with the team in reflective sessions illuminated how pleased the team were about his progress and how appreciative Luke appeared of being able to use the phone to stay in contact with people and watch videos. The team felt relieved that Luke was showing skills in an area that may reduce his risk of relapse and expressed being pleasantly surprised by Luke's engagement in and development through the task.

Summary

Birchwood (2015) cogently makes the case that CBT-P has become a very complex intervention and, because the population is heterogeneous, it risks losing impact because the effect on individual mechanisms and outcomes is diluted. Here, we have been very clear: our focus is on behaviour and distress. These are the key barriers to personal recovery. Birchwood et al. (2017) have further argued that the next generation of CBT-P should be more clearly targeted to avoid getting lost in the scattershot of complex packages of care. What is required, they argue, is a paradigm of theoretical development, leading to targeted intervention focused on the mechanism of interest. This is precisely our aim through our theoretical paradigm CARM. Our mechanism of interest is in-situation beliefs. Additionally, we mobilise the full resources of the team to deliver CBT-P interventions in a timely, highly targeted manner guided by EWS-R.

Chapter 9

Intervening Across Internal and External Domains of the Person's World

Introduction

In Chapter 8, we discussed the use of TBCT and the ways this can be used with teams to target barriers to recovery for service users. Also, Chapter 7 has demonstrated how PBS plans can be derived from our SAFE formulation process and used to redefine the context of problematic behaviour by reinforcing socially acceptable means of achieving the same behavioural function. In the original SAFE approach (Meaden & Hacker, 2010), interventions for what we now term active and passive behaviours largely focused on behavioural interventions. We initially drew on behavioural interventions best exemplified through the literature on people with learning disabilities. However, the past decade has taught us that to deliver these well requires considerable consistency by the team which is not always feasible. Another issue is of generalisability. Whilst behavioural interventions delivered in inpatient type settings may be effective (e.g. Leff & Szmidla, 2002), these may not generalise into the community. Moreover, those in community settings may struggle to effectively offer such interventions. SAFE was always designed as a broad framework based on need-adapted principles (Alanen, 1997), and here we discuss how we have expanded the range of approaches we incorporate into our work.

To further advance our understanding of potential intervention strategies, this chapter will build on the distinction highlighted in our CARM formulation between internal and external factors and consider interventions for distress and problematic risk behaviour across setting events, triggers and reinforcers (see Chapter 5). This CARM formulation structure is a useful shorthand for organising the approach discussed in this chapter; however, this can easily be translated to other formulation structures, for example the cognitive ABC formulation discussed in Chapter 3, (see also Figure 6.3, Chapter 6).

Internal and External Factors

As we have already discussed in Chapter 6, within the CARM formulation, setting events build the motivational drive for the risk behaviour, increasing the likelihood that the behaviour will occur in the presence of the trigger (i.e. they

DOI: 10.4324/9781003082811-10

act alongside vulnerability factors as establishing operations; Cipani, 2018). In Chapter 6 we also saw that within the CARM formulation, establishing operations and reinforcers can be understood as either internal or external to the person, with internal factors being somewhat more difficult to accurately identify in the absence of engagement. In this chapter, for clarity of explanation, we will typically present these as separate; however, it is important to note that in some cases, the distinction between internal and external events may be somewhat arbitrary, and it is not unusual for these to be present in ways that may influence each other.

Case Illustration: Reggie

Reggie presents with paranoid and antisocial personality traits and a history of gang-related violence (vulnerability factors). He visited a new inpatient unit, and in this stressful situation the unfamiliar unit (external setting event) was associated with jumping to conclusions and paranoid, hostile interpretations of other's motives and behaviours (internal setting events). In the presence of ambiguous and unusual peer behaviours such as talking to unseen voices (external trigger), Reggie felt high levels of anxiety, anger and threat (internal trigger) which increased his risk of violence (shouting at and threatening other service users and staff).

In Reggie's case, we can understand that the external setting events and triggers (a new unit, odd behaviours from others), in the context of internal setting events and triggers (paranoid interpretations, threat and anger), helped to establish the function of violence through an interacting process. This illustrates how it is often important to understand how the internal and external factors of the CARM formulation may be hypothesised to interact, as this will provide clues about how best to plan suitable interventions. In Reggie's case, for example familiarising him with the unit gradually through graded leave (intervention focussed on the setting events) reduced the chances of him misunderstanding the other service users' behaviour, and this was used alongside offering him a place to retreat to when he became agitated and upset (intervention focussed on triggers) to reduce the frequency of the violent threats to others. Longer-term interventions may include supporting Reggie to develop his emotional regulation skills alongside interpersonal or social skills training (i.e. expanding his repertoire for managing the triggers).

When developing formulations and interventions, it is important to understand the impact of the challenging or risk behaviours on the person's well-being, quality of life and recovery. Understanding the service user's values can help with this, which we discuss later, alongside broader assessments of outcomes that are personally meaningful (which we discuss in more detail in Chapter 11).

Internally Focussed Interventions

Internally focused interventions can be distributed across setting events, triggers and reinforcing factors; in our experience there is not a single set pattern, and some techniques may work across all three areas. However, where these tend to be focussed at one factor in the CARM formulation more than another we have identified this in our descriptions.

Targeting Beliefs

Perhaps, some of the most powerful psychological interventions directed primarily at the internal level are those designed to modify cognitive appraisals. This can usually be understood as the setting events or "B" in our ABC model, bearing in mind the distinction we have drawn between pan-situational and in-situation beliefs (Meaden et al., 2015). As discussed in previous chapters, we take the view that pan-situational beliefs are those operating across a wide variety of situations whereas in-situation beliefs are the more immediate drivers of distress and problematic behaviours in a given situation or context. Generally, to achieve long-term change, cognitive therapy tends to be focussed on modification of pan-situational beliefs as these are hypothesised to underpin a range of distressing emotions, experiences and behaviours and include psychotic beliefs (e.g. Chadwick et al., 1996; Chadwick, 2006). However, for many service users with whom our teams work, such pan-situational beliefs show poor response to therapeutic approaches and are not the immediate drivers of distress and problematic behaviour. For these reasons, we tend to focus on in-situation beliefs for cognitive-behavioural interventions targeted at the "internal" domain. This may include those interventions that are encompassed within TBCT (see Chapter 8). There are some complementary approaches for working with in-situation beliefs that we have found particularly helpful when using the SAFE approach, which we describe next.

Behavioural Experiments

Behavioural experiments (Bennett-Levy et al., 2004) are a good opportunity to test out logical consequences of in-situation beliefs while at the same time offering an opportunity to practise graded exposure, for example to feared stimuli. This offers an opportunity to test out the predicted consequences of a set of expectations in order to re-evaluate these in light of the outcome of an agreed behavioural experiment (e.g. *I ignored the voices' command and nothing bad happened*). Well-constructed behavioural experiments can offer an opportunity to modify beliefs; however, it is imperative that such interventions are developed within the context of a strong therapeutic relationship. Many of our service users have strongly held convictions in fearful appraisals such as paranoid interpretations and to question and test these out requires courage and faith within the therapeutic process. As such, time can be very well invested in developing strong, trusting relationships and slowly building up to the questioning of such deeply held and, from the service users' point of view, protective beliefs. Furthermore, avoidance (a common safety behaviour) may be seen as a way of surviving the feared consequences (which may be perceived as life-threatening) and as such, motivational enhancement (Westra et al., 2011) or values-based work can be key to developing motivation for change.

Identifying Values to Facilitate Change

To support behavioural change with service users, we have found that it can often be helpful to build awareness of important life goals or motivations that may be compromised due to problematic cognitions. Acceptance and Commitment Therapy (ACT) is one approach we have found useful to draw upon here, with its emphasis on values as part of a wider, behaviourally focussed set of interventions. ACT has a developing evidence base in people with psychosis (Jansen et al., 2020). It is considered a transdiagnostic approach, with many techniques and approaches used to harness behavioural change, regardless of the diagnosis, and including groups whose needs can make them hard to reach (Villanueva et al., 2019). By identifying values that are important to a person, attention can be drawn to beliefs, feelings or behaviours that limit or block movement towards goals that are consistent with these. Often, movement towards valued life goals comes with the anticipated (temporary) cost of increased discomfort or distress, and by drawing attention to how avoidance leads to unfulfilled goals, motivation can be developed for testing out beliefs that underpin the distress. Teaching emotional regulation strategies so that distress can be managed more effectively is key in such an approach. ACT includes mindfulness-based approaches – which have demonstrated efficacy in people with distressing psychosis (Chadwick, 2006; Jansen et al., 2020).

Changing the Way the Person Relates to Their Experiences

A key aspect of so-called third wave behavioural approaches such as ACT is the focus on changing the relationship that the person has with their experience. Rather than getting caught up in experiential avoidance or rumination, people can learn to notice their experiences as transitory aspects of their lived world, often through the practice of mindful attention (Chadwick, 2006). This can be particularly helpful when combined with an awareness of individual values, facilitating an exploration of what is important for the person and how habitual responses (such as avoidance) might be limiting the expression of value-consistent action.

Case Study: Rizzi

Rizzi believes that the world around her is populated by evil demons, and that these evil entities can take any form and use various powers to persecute and torment her. Rizzi fears going outside, as trips out are filled with fear, dread and hypervigilance to internal symptoms. Innocuous sensations become interpreted as signs that the demons are starting to plague her, which leads to rumination, panic and avoidance. Panic attacks are taken as evidence of the power of the demons' control over her, and avoidance of the outside is reinforced through removal of the anticipatory anxiety. Rizzi spends most of her time inside, rarely leaving the house or her room; however, she would like to spend time with her family who live locally (connectedness with others being a key value) and continuing a culinary course she started before her most recent relapse (again linked to her value of connectedness).

Rizzi was open to discussions and self-reports of her feelings. She reported 100% conviction in the belief that the demons were persecuting her and that she was powerless to reduce their influence over her experiences. Rizzi reported high levels of "stress" and was open to looking at ways of trying to manage this. Through the practice of mindful attention, Rizzi became familiar with the patterns of "stress" and "anxiety" she felt in her body and noted that she could reduce these using mindfulness techniques. Mindfulness practice and psychoeducation regarding anxiety and the nature of the mind (metacognitive insight; Chadwick, 2006, 2014) were used to explore aspects of Rizzi's experiences gently and openly, and she noticed some of the habitual patterns of her mind, such as a tendency to ruminate. As Rizzi's confidence in the therapeutic process and her ability to respond mindfully to distress grew, attention was drawn to the ways in which avoidance was preventing her from fully realising some of her values (e.g. connectedness with her family). Behavioural experiments were designed, supporting Rizzi to leave the house, using her new-found mindfulness skills. Graded practice was used to help her get on the train using these skills, at first accompanied and eventually on her own, until she was able to visit her family.

Rizzi reported that the demons still tormented her. However, she described how she used her skills to respond to the demons mindfully, and found that, often, she was able to "keep them at bay" until she had achieved the activity she wanted, such as visiting her family or doing her shopping on her own. At last contact, Rizzi had restarted her culinary course.

In this example we can see how careful exploration with Rizzi into her internal world, guided by evidence-based principles of mindfulness and CBT for psychosis was able to create space for her to learn new ways of responding to her distressing experiences. Her interpretations of these were never directly challenged, and indeed, we see no evidence that they ever changed – she still believed these were caused by demons – but Rizzi increased her awareness of her ability to manage these differently, created flexibility in her behavioural responses and was able to enhance her well-being through committed, value-based action.

Cognitive Processing and Behaviour

There is now well-established evidence of cognitive difficulties in people who have received a schizophrenia diagnosis, although the nature of these appears to be rather heterogeneous (Habtewold et al., 2020). As such, it is important to consider the role of possible cognitive problems in problematic behaviour and distress. Fundamental cognitive processing deficits, such as slow processing, are important to identify, so that modifications and adaptations to the environment (external interventions) can be made or coping skills enhanced. There is some evidence that approaches to cognitive training such as cognitive remediation therapy may offer some help in this area; however, it remains unclear what factors limit its effectiveness (Reser et al., 2019). Suggested factors that may limit the benefits observed in this treatment include premorbid IQ, baseline cognition and task progress.

It is our experience that rather than focussing on general cognitive deficits, it is the social cognitive difficulties that show more promise for meaningful change when working with our service user group. There is evidence that difficulties in processing social information is most closely associated with functional outcome (Fett et al., 2011; Javed & Charles, 2018), and so supporting these may be most likely to lead to meaningful changes for the service user. We have found it useful to use the model described by Couture et al. (2006), which offers a basic heuristic for understanding the broad areas of social cognitive deficits that may be problematic in our service users. Key areas of deficits can include, but are not limited to, theory of mind, emotion recognition, jumping to conclusions and attribution biases (Couture et al., 2006; Fox & Harrop, 2015).

Given that social cognitive information is necessarily complex and dynamic, we have found that video-based approaches seem to have more real-world validity in helping to assess service user's needs and provide training. The Awareness of Social Inference Test (McDonald, 2012) has proven particularly useful as it allows for the recognition of specific emotions as well as theory of mind tasks, while training can be achieved by reviewing the videos in sessions. Linked to this, use of video clips from common TV shows (such as The Simpsons character, "Comic Book Guy") has proven a good source of examples of sarcasm. These can be used to illustrate and discuss social situations whilst also being entertaining and enhancing the therapeutic relationship with service users.

Particular therapeutic approaches in this area include Social Cognitive Interaction Training (Roberts et al., 2016) and Metacognitive Training (Moritz et al., 2013). There is a developing evidence base for such social cognitive training (Horan & Green, 2019); however, these are generally designed to be run in group settings (the natural format for such sessions) which may complicate matters for our service users who have very specific social-cognitive needs or may be too suspicious to join a group. In these cases, individual work can continue using the same approaches, although some extra thought needs to be given to practising and generalising any learning outside of individual therapeutic sessions. This is the advantage of adopting a team approach whereby other members of the team can be utilised. Perhaps somewhat unsurprisingly for this service user group, our experience suggests that takeaway tasks benefit from being socially supported and scaffolded if they are to have any form of success.

Case Study: Darren

Darren, while living in a low-secure inpatient unit, showed a tendency to jump to conclusions about other people's motives. It was hypothesised that this was maintained by some emotional processing deficits, such that Darren generally concludes (incorrectly) that people have negative intentions towards him (also an attribution bias). In regular sessions, Darren was encouraged to review video clips from The Awareness of Social Inference Test and was surprised to learn that he generally viewed most people as "angry" or "upset" regardless of their true emotions. Reviewing the tapes allowed Darren to pause each clip and discuss key aspects to help him review his answers. Darren spent time supported by staff members he trusted, carrying out key tasks on the unit (e.g. asking for his evening meal, making other requests, volunteering for house jobs), discussing his interpretations of the interactions he was having and what he based his interpretation on – the "clues" from the other person. This offered Darren an opportunity to practise emotional processing skills as well as monitor his attributional tendencies. Over time, Darren accepted a "stop and think" card to carry in his pocket, which reminded him to "stop" when he was making a judgement about others' motivations and "think" about the evidence he was using to make this judgement.

In the case of Darren, we can see the benefits of having access to a 24-hour supported care environment, as Darren could be encouraged to make use of experimenting with developing skills and knowledge supported by those he trusted. This also increased the "dosage", or the number of learning opportunities open to Darren, which in turn increased the speed and effectiveness of the intervention. Clearly, this could be dovetailed neatly with a TBCT intervention (Chapter 8) mobilising the whole team resource to support Darren in practising his skills throughout his daily encounters.

Social Skills Training

A related but separate factor to cognitive tendencies and deficits is that of social skill. Social skill deficits have long been noted in people diagnosed with schizophrenia. Social skills training was among some of the earliest of the evidence-based psychological interventions to be developed for people with psychosis (Benton & Schroeder, 1990; Eisler et al., 1978). There are well-established protocols for social skills training and readers are directed to the seminal work by Bellack et al. (2004) in this regard. However, there are some adaptations that may need to be considered when working with hard-to-reach populations. For instance, social skill deficits may also be linked to lack of opportunity to access typically desired social situations due to repeated lengthy hospitalisations or institutionalisation that can unfortunately follow from prolonged inpatient stays. New opportunities to develop and practice social skills are therefore of key importance and care should be given to plan the sorts of discharge packages likely to be available for each service user, with training tailored for the environment that they are likely to find themselves in. For example it may be decided that making positive requests from the service staff may be of most immediate benefit and prioritised above the skill of discussing financial transactions in shops, if, in this instance, the service user has limited leave or limited access to their finances. However, if the same service user is looking to regain leave or access to their finances, then the reverse may be true. It is also possible that cognitive difficulties may make the acquisition or retention of new information difficult, and so training should be adapted to meet any such needs (e.g. use of handouts, repetition, structured recall and reminders, backward chaining; Meaden & Hacker, 2010). We would emphasise that focusing on observed positives and aiming for "errorless" learning can be useful in reducing perceived stigma and fostering hope in service users, alongside having realistic aims and steps to the training process. Furthermore, the backward chaining of steps of a new skill can usefully harness the intrinsic rewards of task completion (Meaden & Hacker, 2010).

Awareness and Management of Emotions

Strong emotions can often be observed to act as triggers to problematic behaviour and may in themselves be distressing (e.g. avoidance and anxiety; violence and anger). Removal or discharge of feelings can then act as reinforcers for behaviour to reoccur. Emotion recognition and healthy management of such emotions are therefore a key area for interventions.

Emotional knowledge and recognition have already been discussed in the preceding section on social cognition. Similarly, we have discussed the role of anxiety and the various interventions that can be used to deal with avoidance (a reinforcer) and the in-situation beliefs that underpin this (setting events). It is our experience, however, that gaining emotional knowledge is an important step in equipping service users with effective strategies for managing problematic emotions such as anxiety before further intervention continues. This can build hope for change, model the effectiveness of personal coping strategies and enhance engagement. There is renewed interest in coping strategy enhancement (Hayward et al., 2018) alongside increased awareness of the effective therapeutic targets for people with schizophrenia diagnoses including worry and avoidance (Freeman et al., 2019). Bernard et al. (2015) describe a formulation-driven cognitive-behavioural approach to dealing with emotional dysfunction, including the assessment of emotional regulation.

The key when dealing with distressing emotions is often to be clear which emotions service users are struggling with and adapting support accordingly. Common areas of need include strong feelings of being threatened (fear, anxiety, worry), of being unfairly treated (frustration, anger) or of feeling like there is little hope (sadness, hopeless, worthless); such feelings may (or may not) be linked to symptomatic distress, such as that associated with "poor me" or "bad me" paranoia (Trower & Chadwick, 1995). Where there is a clear pattern of emotions, then tailoring the emotional coping repertoire is likely to be more helpful than relying on more generic approaches. A technique that can be usefully borrowed from the compassion-focussed therapy approach is that of a "compassionate kitbag" (Lucre & Clapton, 2021). This is a method for developing a set of compassionate ways of being in the world (towards self and others) and often takes the form of a physical container (e.g. a decorated box or even an empty shoebox) that can be filled with objects that in themselves are considered soothing (e.g. a familiar smell or an image) or represents a technique that can be used in a compassionate manner (e.g. a seaside pebble to represent the notion that all things change; an image of a lotus flower to represent mindfulness practice). In our experience, such an approach allows the collection of a useful set of tools and tips (beyond abstract words on a page), supports the initiation of behavioural action towards self-care and compassion, increases self-efficacy for self-management and acts as a physical reminder of the importance of action in this area.

Considerations for Internal Factors Linked to "Passive Behaviours"

Traditionally, CBT-P has focussed on the appraisals and reinforcers that underpin positive symptoms and associated risk behaviours; however, there is a developing evidence base for the value of CBT for "negative symptoms" (Fox & Meaden, 2015, see also Chapter 8). Many of the techniques already discussed in this chapter are also useful for these "passive behaviours", albeit with a few modifications (e.g. Chapter 8). Many of the enduring problematic behaviours that the staff struggle to understand and manage include those that would be considered passive behaviours. As discussed in Chapter 8, passive behaviours can be understood as being at least partly maintained by negative expectations – low expectancies for pleasure; low expectancies for success; low expectancies for acceptance; perception of limited resources (Fox & Meaden, 2015; Rector et al., 2005). Often associated with these negative expectancies is an amotivational state typically identified in people with "negative symptoms", described by Foussias and Remington (2010) as a lack in the appetitive drive alongside an intact consummatory drive (i.e. "wanting" is reduced while "liking" remains). This means that although people may not expect positive outcomes from their activity (the reduced appetitive drive) they retain the capacity to enjoy them (the consummatory system), which indicates the value of behavioural experiments and other exposure- and learning-based interventions for passive behaviours. Using such approaches to test out negative expectancies and gently highlighting discrepancies between expectations and reality, alongside exposure to enjoyable activities, can be useful ways of targeting internal factors that maintain such passive behaviours.

Similarly, identifying important values can be an excellent starting point when working with passive behaviours. When asked, many people will initially identify goals that are difficult to obtain, so when working with passive behaviours, identifying underpinning values can be a helpful way of ensuring that lack of obtaining the goal is not experienced as evidence for lack of success (a negative expectancy). Values, by their nature, point the direction rather than serve as the destination, so can act as a safe way of discussing service user achievements without running such a risk of exposing them to fear of failure.

A meta-analysis has offered some initial support for the notion that skills development and behavioural activation are key to the (modest) effectiveness of psychosocial interventions for passive behaviours (Lutgens et al., 2017). We have already discussed in this chapter how skills training can be built into intervention strategies for internal factors, but again, care should be taken to properly assess and where necessary to formulate these as distinct from skill deficits that may be linked to concurrent positive symptoms.

Externally Focussed Interventions

Using reinforcement remains an important strand of our intervention processes. Our CARM formulation explicitly attempts to identify the reinforcers of problem behaviours. Early reinforcement-based behavioural interventions can be found in work employing Token Economies, which aimed to use these principles to reinforce desired behaviour by providing tokens (that may later be exchanged for naturalistic reinforcers) contingent upon the presentation of specified target behaviours. Tokens were used to bridge the delay in the expression of the target behaviour and the provision of the contingent reinforcement. These approaches were often used in large psychiatric institutions to help rehabilitate those with chronic psychosis by encouraging the expression of socially desirable behaviours such as ward work and social skills as well as improve self-care (Ayllon & Azrin, 1965). These approaches fell out of favour since they were implemented broadly across settings and did not take into account the function of the individual's behaviour. We continue to draw on behavioural reinforcement principles in our intervention planning; however, this is underpinned by an understanding of the function of the behaviour for individuals alongside the wider context within which behaviour occurs (internal and external factors). Furthermore, this chapter has illustrated the importance of offering interventions that may help correct the mismatch between the external environment and the person's interpretation of this, through the processes discussed earlier. However, this is not always desirable, possible or necessary, for example due to poor engagement or the self-protective function of a delusion (e.g. "poor me" paranoia; Trower & Chadwick, 1995). An important and what we would consider overarching external factor for consideration and potential intervention is that of quality of life and well-being. The recovery literature has highlighted the importance of recovery in the presence of mental health needs and how the pursuit of a meaningful life is itself an important factor in well-being (Papadopoulos et al., 2013). As such, external factors are important components of the lifeworld of the service user that can contribute to distress and problematic behaviour, and these can often be feasible areas for meaningful intervention either on their own or in conjunction with internal factors.

The key to interventions is to consider the quality of the service user's life and how the environment may be modified to improve their well-being through changes to external setting events, triggers and reinforcers. Modification of these aspects of the service user's lifeworld may be more within the capability of services than modification of internal factors, and it is our experience that these can be a good place to start when planning interventions in order to initiate helpful change quickly and effectively. Indeed, it is our experience that once the environment is a better fit for the service user's well-being, further intervention (e.g. on internal factors, such as in-situational beliefs) may no longer be necessary – in which case these interventions can be considered the most ethically appropriate.

Mobilisation of the resources required to properly formulate, understand and modify the environmental contexts that contribute to well-being is complex yet critical. Here, we suggest that the MDT is key not just to understand the complexity of our service user's environment (such as inpatient services and community teams) but also in accessing the power to implement changes in that environment. For example in our earlier case of Reggie and the paranoid aggressive interpretations of other service user's actions, involvement of the consultant psychiatrist and nursing management was crucial in first grading his leave and exposure to the new environment and, second, identifying somewhere safe Reggie could retreat to in order to help regulate his anger. These interventions, although conceptually simple, were grounded upon a thorough understanding of the internal and external contexts to his lifeworld (a CARM formulation developed by the MDT) and facilitated through access to the necessary resources required to implement effective changes.

Assessment

Our SLF can be a useful starting point for developing an initial understanding of possible external barriers to social participation, well-being and recovery for the service user. The common areas discussed in teams we have worked with include:

- Detention under the Mental Health Act;
- Dislocation from family and friends;

- Impoverished support networks;
- Limitations in the local environment (e.g. lack of single sex amenities);
- Restricted access to the community.

It is easy to see how, although some limitations may be imposed for risk management, such restrictions often have negative implications for the service user's life. Understanding how external limitations may link to impairments in aspects of the life of the service user is therefore important. To achieve this, it can be helpful to use well-being or quality-of-life tools that identify different domains that may be important to different individuals. We use a Quality-of-Life Card Sort tool that explores a range of activities and whether these are "liked" or "disliked" by a service user and whether these are "present" or "absent". Items where there is a discrepancy (e.g. liked items that are absent) can then be discussed, and if these are personally important for the service user, these can potentially be introduced into the person's life. Similarly, the ACT-based Value Conversations cards (Hayes & Coyne, 2021) are a set of images and words on cards that service users can sort through and explain which are meaningful for them; these can be used to develop interventions focussed on access to values that may have been impaired or restricted.

Choice, Control and Autonomy

In a small meta-synthesis, Shepherd et al. (2016) identified a role for personal autonomy in the recovery of service users within forensic mental health settings. Our experience suggests that for many of our service users, control and choice can be severely limited. This may be due to restrictions imposed as part of risk management. However, it can also be important to look at ways of trying to express alternative ways of meeting the need for choice and control. We have found that it can be helpful to reflect with the team on the limitations the service may impose on service users' freedoms, and how these can be used to understand some of the seemingly "unreasonable" requests from them. We might invite them, for example to consider how they would feel if they could not get a cup of coffee when they wanted one.

Case Study: Anwar

Anwar is a 35-year-old male residing in a CRU. He was reported to make many requests from the staff at short notice and would become impatient when these needs were not met, becoming verbally aggressive and threatening towards the staff. Anwar reported that the staff were being "spiteful" in their restrictions, such as not allowing him to order a fast-food takeaway every evening. When his SLF was reviewed, it was noted that there were few areas where Anwar could express a sense of control. Anwar was often in bed when the meal choices were offered for the evening, so he would miss out on making his choices, and he was unable to watch his favourite TV show due to another service user taking control of the TV remote from early in the day. Anwar's family were unable to visit due to COVID-19 pandemic restrictions, and as they did not have access to digital resources required for the remote video calls, he had not seen them in over six months (when previously they visited every week). Anwar had also not been able to go out to buy any more clothes due to the pandemic restrictions, but as he was unable to go out, he did not believe the team's claims that the shops were closed.

It was agreed that should Anwar miss the opportunity to choose his evening meal, then he would either be supported to make his own meal in the evening or he would be able to choose his meal in preparation for the next day. Anwar was supported to look online with staff support to buy some of his preferred clothes, and he was also supported to initiate talking to his family weekly on the phone (in the absence of any visits to the unit). The staff on the CRU arranged a rota for the television to help Anwar and others to have an opportunity to watch their favourite TV shows and make access to the TV more equitable amongst the service users. The frequency of the verbal aggression from Anwar as measured by the START severity scales decreased on days where the staff team were able to follow the agreed guidelines. Ongoing monitoring of the plans alongside a PBS plan were used to help Anwar express his frustrations in a more appropriate manner.

Environment and Adaptations

It may be that where internal factors limit the abilities of the service user (e.g. cognitive deficits), then there may be a requirement for external interventions to manage these. This may include, for example reminders or prompts from the staff in case of service users with memory deficits. Such adaptations can make allowances for the needs of service users that cannot be met by internally focussed interventions. Clearly, where there are physical impairments (e.g. difficulties with mobility) these should be addressed not only as part of meeting routine health and social care needs but also in an attempt to understand potential contributions to challenging behaviour (e.g. de Winter et al., 2011). Ensuring that the environment is a good match for the person's needs is, of course, a core component of good quality care and should not be overlooked when seeking to understand distress and challenging behaviour.

Other aspects of the environment that can have a significant impact on recovery include access to suitable living conditions and necessary resources. Housing, social networks and social capital are all important factors associated with well-being and health outcomes for all people (Cattell, 2001) and are no less important for service users. Access to factors such as quality housing and social connectedness are therefore important external factors to consider regarding mental health and well-being (Cattell, 2001; Hare-Duke et al., 2019; Saeri et al., 2018). Although these can be complex to navigate and influence, there is increasing evidence that doing so can have an important impact on quality of life (e.g. Wakefield et al., 2020). These factors are particularly important to consider when working with service users in the community or thinking about those approaching discharge from inpatient services.

Perhaps, a more immediate external factor for consideration is the range of stimuli in the environment. There is evidence that a "low arousal" approach can be helpful for reducing distress and challenging behaviours (McDonnell et al., 1998; McDonnell, 1999). This can involve the management of the environment to reduce identified high arousal stimuli (e.g. increasing physical space between people, reducing eye contact) but also supporting the staff to access the individual resources to enable such work alongside enhancing the local culture and general approach to challenging behaviours. As well as TBCT and regular staff supervision sessions, we also advocate regular training to ensure that new members of the team quickly become socialised into the SAFE model of care.

Staff Training and Support

Team member attitudes and the relationship with the service user have been consistently identified as key when considering recovery in forensic mental health services (Simpson & Penney, 2018). It is all too easy to be blind to potential triggers within our own teams that may lead to distress and problematic behaviour, such that team supervision and training is essential to notice this, prevent burnout and reduce unhelpful interactional styles. TBCT can be used to identify unhelpful assumptions that may underpin such styles (Chapter 8). Of course, sometimes interactions may not be immediately modifiable, such as when they involve other service users, and so identification of any problematic relationships between service users and the development of ways of carefully helping users to manage these (or avoid each other) can be helpful.

Given some of the factors discussed in the previous sections, such as social cognitive deficits around attributional styles and jumping to conclusions, a key area for external focus is the personal interactions around the service user (e.g. staff, family). Ongoing training and support are likely to be required to maintain changes in staff team behaviour and prevent the return to any previously learnt (habitual) ways of responding, particularly when services are stressed or under pressure. Of course, it is also important to ensure that team members are looked after and cared for themselves, particularly due to the links between work-related stress and challenging behaviours. Schablon et al. (2012) and Ballatt and Campling (2011) describe the complexities of working in healthcare, the consequences that can result from toxic care systems that, for example alienate staff from patients and potential ways of managing services in ways that reduce burn-out and improve the quality of care.

A systemic factor that can also be key is the availability of staff who know and have a relationship with the service user. As we have already noted, relationships are crucial for the delivery of high-quality therapeutic interventions, and this is unlikely to be possible in the case of high staff turnover and reliance on agency or "bank" staff. A stable core staff team is a prerequisite for the delivery of SAFE, and the absence of this can usually be considered an external setting event or trigger for problematic behaviour or distress.

Social Networks

Beyond the confines of care services, the transition from institutional to community networks needs to be carefully considered. When entering services, it is important to recognise the potential dislocation of service users from their social networks such as families and friends. Whilst networks may not always appear supportive, it is important to acknowledge the relevance of social networks in recovery – including the move from institutional networks such as staff teams back to those found in the community (Shepherd et al., 2016; Simpson & Penney, 2018). When considering social networks, mapping them can be a useful exercise in understanding who is around and the nature of their relationship with the service user. Care maps have recently been explored in people with long-term health conditions to shed light on the service user's social lifeworld (Young et al., 2021). For service users with problematic substance misuse, interventions such as Social Behaviour and Network Therapy (Copello et al., 2006) focus on the mobilisation of social networks supportive of positive behavioural change.

Summary

In this chapter, we have seen how a range of evidence-based interventions can be accessed and mobilised in order to understand and manage factors associated with problematic behaviours and distress. The distinction identified in the CARM formulation between internal and external factors is a useful approach to orienting the focus of the care team to the broad nature of the factors involved in the maintenance of problematic behaviour and distress. Psychological evidence can be used to develop the understanding of these factors through bespoke assessment and formulation and interventions designed accordingly.

The function of the behaviour for the service user is a key feature of this approach, and it is important to understand the internal and external contexts within which behaviour occurs to develop effective formulations and appropriate interventions. We have seen that a range of complementary psychological approaches can be used to achieve this understanding and to develop interventions that enhance recovery and well-being, integrated around the notion of more effective functional behaviour. Whilst these may draw upon a variety of psychological evidence, the SAFE (and specifically the CARM) approach guides how these are integrated into an understanding of factors that are hypothesised to maintain difficulties for service users and suggests potential interventions. For example by understanding Reggie's feelings of threat (trigger) when in an unfamiliar and unpredictable environment (setting events) in the context of past use of violence in gangs (vulnerability factor), we can start to develop support plans for the immediate term (graded exposure to reduce unfamiliarity; having a safe place to retreat to) whilst also developing plans for longer-term interventions (interpersonal training, emotional regulation skills). This increases Reggie's ability to manage the distress more effectively and act in ways that enhance his well-being (e.g. effective risk self-management, greater freedoms). This illustrates how different approaches can be deployed in the service of personally meaningful behavioural change and reduction in distress as part of enabling recovery. Understanding what matters to the person is a key component of such an approach, as subjective well-being and quality of life can only be truly defined and understood by the individual who is experiencing them. This again underlines the importance of the multidisciplinary shared team approach to providing care, as part of enhancing the ability of the team to build relationships with people who can be hard to reach and help.

Although in this chapter we have discussed internal and external factors as separate, it should be clear that these will commonly overlap and interact and so interventions may realistically need to be developed to target multiple maintaining processes. For example in the case of Anwar discussed in this chapter, intervention was focused on the external environment to reduce his frustration but also on internal targets to train him to express his frustration in more socially acceptable ways. When working with those with such complex needs, it is imperative to remain open and flexible in the development of formulations, so that interventions can be best developed and enhanced in the light of changing evidence and understanding: to be need-adapted.

Chapter 10

Using Multiple Shared Formulations to Inform Care Planning and Intervention

Introduction

Since the initial work on SAFE we have found that our original approach to care planning (Meaden & Hacker, 2010) using GAST (Kiresuk et al., 1994) was simply too complex for the majority of the staff to engage in. We have described in detail in Chapter 7 how we utilise and have integrated PBS plans into the SAFE approach. However, not all of the information obtained from our four of the five areas (described later) readily lend themselves to PBS plans. We have found that a range of care planning processes and templates is needed to fully support the range of care plans that can result from a shared assessment and formulation process. Having completed the various assessment tools and processes and formulated individual risk and problem behaviours, the team will have a wealth of information upon which to base their care plans. In this chapter, we describe how we utilise this information from the broader START process and our other formulations to prioritise and plan other types of care plan.

Care Planning Sources

In SAFE we utilise information from five key sources in our care planning process. Each of these yields a number potential broad and specific care planning recovery goals.

1 RGPI:

    (a) Personal goals
    (b) Agreed barriers to recovery.

2 SLF:

    (a) Internal barriers
    (b) External barriers
    (c) Social participation goals
    (d) Building on strengths
    (e) Three key barriers.

DOI: 10.4324/9781003082811-11

3 START:

    (a) Key item strengths and vulnerabilities

    (b) Critical items strengths and vulnerabilities

    (c) THREAT items.

4 CARM:

    (a) Setting events and EWS-R (active behaviours)

    (b) Expectancy beliefs (passive behaviours)

    (c) Triggers

    (d) Reinforcers.

5 Static-Dynamic Risk Formulation:

    (a) Dynamic stable factors

    (b) Dynamic acute factors.

An important caveat when care planning in SAFE is to return to our need-adapted treatment principles (Meaden & Hacker, 2010). Critically, care plans should not contradict or overlap with each other and they should take account of the changing needs and be reviewed regularly. In the following sections, we look at how information gained from four of these five areas (CARM care plans having been covered extensively in previous chapters) can be care planned.

Care Planning Using Four Key Sources

Here, we use two key case studies to illustrate how we can utilise the significant amount of information and shared understanding derived from the SAFE process. We return again to our case studies, Steve introduced in Chapter 5 and Otis who featured in Chapter 6.

Case Study: Steve

Steve has a long history of criminal behaviour and violent assaults and has a number of pro-criminal associates from when he was involved in gang culture. Steve was married for four years, and throughout this relationship there was a lot of domestic abuse. Steve has a history of violent behaviours towards others, including gang-related violence. Steve moreover has a history of smoking cannabis (e.g. positive drug screens) but has always denied doing so. Steve denies having a mental illness and struggles to acknowledge any changes in his mental state. Steve often claims that his family are out to steal from him and harm him and has been known to physically attack family members and throw furniture around the house. Many of the incidents of violence can be attributed to poor control of psychotic symptoms such as paranoia; however, Steve also expresses mistrust of authority and pro-criminal attitudes (e.g. *"you need to put them down before they get to you, and when they go down, you better make sure they stay down"*). His most recent offence involved attacking a policeman (he was intoxicated at the time); he was arrested and later sent to prison. Whilst in prison, his mental health deteriorated and he started developing delusional ideas that it was his ex-wife who sent him to prison and that she was sending gangs to hurt him and his family. Steve expressed the belief that the prison wardens were also involved in this conspiracy and were making threats to harm him through the use of special codes. He heard voices telling him that he and his family were in danger and reported that he was able to receive messages from the radio and TV, "tuning into" conversations between the prison staff and gangs outside of prison. Steve was subsequently transferred to a medium forensic psychiatric hospital under Section 37/41. Steve was stabilised on a regular medication monitoring regime and was eventually stepped down to a locked rehabilitation unit.

Addressing these multiple risks required multiple levels of formulation-informed care planning. When the staff talked to Steve about his risk history, he initially blamed others and claimed that he was provoked or that he did not remember the incident. Steve tended to either deny or minimise his behaviours.

Information From Steve's SAFE Process

1   Steve's RGPI

Steve completed the RGPI with his named nurse with whom he had formed a good relationship. They identified a number of goals:

   (a) Learning to manage his money better
   (b) To manage his medication on his own
   (c) To attend the gym and go to Muay Thai or boxing classes
   (d) To be discharged to his own accommodation
   (e) To find work.

The following barriers were noted to achieving these goals:

(a) Unwanted physical contact with his peers in the forms and pretending to punch them
(b) Shouting loudly at his peers to scare them

(c) Visiting venues and places not agreed prior to his leave

(d) Stealing food and cigarettes from peers and sometimes trading these on the unit.

2 Steve's SLF

In a subsequent reflective practice meeting the team completed an SLF as shown in Table 10.1.

Table 10.1 Steve's SLF

Service Level Formulation

Service User Name   Steve Jones   SU Identifier (*information system number*)

Date Completed   SLF Version 1

Symptoms and impairments *What ongoing symptoms (include diagnosis where relevant) impairments and disabilities the person has as a result of their diagnoses?* Diagnosis: paranoid schizophrenia, frustration, tolerance/restless Positive symptoms: • Persecutory beliefs: believes ex-wife has arranged for gang members to attack him • Hears voices • ADHD – impulsive/distractible/poor antisocial and paranoid personality traits • History of criminal behaviour from young age • History of drugs and alcohol use at a young age • Diabetes	**External barriers** *What restrictions and barriers are placed upon the individual externally/from others?* • Section 37/41 of the MHA • Inconsistent staff boundaries/ communication style • No unescorted leave • Family has little contact with Steve
Internal barriers *What does the person do themselves that creates barriers for their recovery?* • Mistrust of others and people in authority • Denial of mental health difficulties • Poor concordance with medication • Stealing food and cigarettes off peers • Trading on the unit • Lacks social boundaries: touching, shouting, juvenile behaviour (pokes, growls, plays practical jokes) • Imitates and mocks the staff and peers • Verbal aggression (swears/insults/threats) • Physical aggression: punching, pulling hair • Poor budgeting skills • Touching/groping others sexually – invading personal space • Not adhering to pre-agreed plans whilst on escorted leave • Denies or minimises risk behaviours • External attribution style – does not take responsibility, does not consider consequences • Antisocial/authoritarian traits	**Participation/ personal recovery** *What does the person want to participate in but is limited due to symptoms, impairments and barriers?* • To manage his medication on his own • To be discharged to his own accommodation • To find work • To join a local gym • To have contact with family (*but due to past assaults they do not want to have contact with Steve*) • To have unescorted leave

Protective factors (*the service users' strength mitigators against relapse and risk*)
• Has good therapeutic alliances with several members of the team (including named nurse)
• Can be reflective when given the space to talk through difficulties that have been identified
• Values praise and positive feedback

Three key recovery barriers (*potential care planning goals*)
• Impulsivity/lack of social boundaries
• Minimises problem behaviours
• Mistrusting/suspicious of others

Table 10.2 Steve's SMART Goal for Community Integration

Steve's SMART goals

Community integration goal:	When?	Who?	Achieved?/ Comments
I want to be able to live safely in the community and stay out of hospital			
Steve to devise a shopping list including where he needs to go for items	By May 2020	OT	Achieved *Coloured Green*
Steve to use his shopping list to practise his shopping trips stick to the agreed places he needs to visit	By June 2020	OT and Nursing Staff (2 to 1)	Achieved *Coloured Green*
Staff to reinforce boundaries if Steve requests to go to other places			
Staff to remind him of his longer-term goal			
Review leave plans as appropriate			
Steve to practise making his own way to the local shops to buy his items	By December 2020	Un-escorted	Not yet *Coloured Red*

It readily became apparent that Steve's barriers to recovery from his RGPI and those identified following his SLF had considerable overlap. This is an important point of reflection that Steve with support could actually identify and acknowledge that these behaviours created barriers for him in his recovery journey even if he subsequently minimised or denied having engaged in such behaviours. Barriers 1 and 3 could be informed by a PBS plan, but not barrier 2. For the remaining behaviour, it was agreed that a simpler care plan could be devised: visiting venues and places not agreed prior to his leave.

A simplified SMART-based template for planning and reviewing such care plan goals (shown in Table 10.2) has been developed (see Chapter 12). This was used here to plan Steve's community leave. The plan is broken down into four SMART steps and forms part of his longer-term goal of community reintegration.

Using this plan, Steve was able to achieve increased leave. However, he continued to require support to avoid transgressing boundaries and consequently was unable to move beyond one-to-one escorted leave. Accordingly, it was agreed to revise the SMART care plan and introduce a further level of escort with a health-care assistant to test out if boundaries could be maintained with a less qualified member of the staff.

1 Steve's START

In agreeing what to target it is helpful to focus on a smaller number of areas and to avoid overlapping and competing efforts (a need-adapted treatment principle, see Meaden & Hacker, 2010). Consideration should be given to how severe and acute current risks are. THREAT (Threats of Harm that are Real, Enactable, Acute and Targeted)-rated items on the START should be prioritised. Some areas will be harder to change, such as antisocial attitudes compared to engagement with recreational activities. It is beneficial for the motivation of both the team and the individual to include areas such as these and especially those where strengths are also evident and can be built upon.

In Table 10.3 we show START items used to identify key and critical items for Steve for potential care planning purposes. A total of 19 out of 20 items were judged as either key strengths or critical vulnerabilities reflecting the high level of needs Steve has and both his risk history and current behaviour on the unit. Table 10.3 shows relevant items used to inform endorsements of key or critical items with intentionally blank areas indicating no strengths or vulnerabilities in that area.

Steve's index offence: hitting a policeman, it was agreed, also remained an area of concern, Steve was still subject to Section 37/41 restrictions from the home office concerning use of alcohol, not associating with pro-criminal peers and compliance with medication. Whilst currently Steve was making progress in all of these areas, the staff were less confident that these would be maintained if unescorted leave was given or following eventual discharge into the community. The historical nature

Table 10.3 Steve's START Items for Key and Critical Areas

START areas	Strengths	Vulnerabilities
Social skills	Pleasant at times Polite at times Joins in group activities sometimes Initiates conversations Good communication skills Socially appropriate behaviour sometimes Feels satisfaction in social situations	Lacks manners at times Immature Intrusive

(Continued)

Table 10.3 (Continued)

START areas	Strengths	Vulnerabilities
Relationships	Superficially gets along with others	Superficial at times Aloof Inconsiderate at times Takes advantage of others Manipulates Provokes Objectifies others Deceptive at times Unfriendly at times Lacks empathy at times
Occupational	Understands the value of education and work Seeks out opportunities at times Is willing to be advised Consents to starting out at a level appropriate to existing experience and skills Reliable at times Sometimes does assignments on time Has good work habits	
Recreational	Aware of recreational opportunities Uses leisure time constructively at times Enjoys recreational activities Plans activities for self and others Takes regular physical exercise	
Self-care	Carries out basic personal hygiene Maintains personal space in satisfactory condition at times Normal sleep patterns Normal eating patterns at times Accepts health teaching at times	Personal hygiene is maintained at less than minimal levels only Dresses in idiosyncratic or inappropriate fashion Does not follow health teaching at times
Mental state		Delusions Hallucinations Flight of idea Impaired attention

(Continued)

Table 10.3 (Continued)

START areas	Strengths	Vulnerabilities
Emotional state	Good spirits at times Sense of humour at times Hopeful at times Ability to experience emotions Mood appropriate to circumstances at times	Depressed at times Labile Pessimistic Feelings of worthlessness at times Hopelessness at times Irritable at times Angry at times
Substance use	Abstains	
Impulse control	Restrained at times Calm at times	Overwrought at times Erratic at times Out-of-control Excited Risk-taking at times Impulsive Acts on spur of moment Does not anticipate consequences Poor frustration tolerance
External triggers		Influenced by disruptive peers Affected by specific destabilisers and changing demands in the environment
Social support	Social support from family and professionals	~~Non-availability or~~ non-acceptance of social support Inadequate social network
Material resources	Adequate means/income No financial drains Stable and satisfactory housing	Irresponsible management of finances
Attitudes		Pro-criminal Callous Remorseless Narcissistic at times Selfish Collusive Hostile at times Dishonest at times Lacks empathy at times Aggressive attributional style Takes offence easily Resentful Self-esteem difficulties

(Continued)

Table 10.3 (Continued)

START areas	Strengths	Vulnerabilities
Medication adherence		Will only accept particular kinds
Rule adherence		Does not attempt to understand the points behind the rules and conditions Disobeys rules at times
Conduct		~~Escapes~~ ~~Barricade~~ Threatens at times Assaults at times Steals Disrupts Sets others up for failure Complains repeatedly about staff without justification at times Insults Teases Intimidates at times Bullies Makes racist, sexist or other such comments Interferes with co-clients' assessments, treatments and management
Insight		Not self-aware Fails to appreciate motivation behind own actions Denies mental, personality or substance use disorder and (if present) the need for interventions Does not identify and/ or manage personal risk factors No recognition of early signs of relapse
Plans	Socially acceptable Realistic at times Focused at times Future-oriented Has plans to achieve short-and long-term goals	

(Continued)

Table 10.3 (Continued)

START areas	Strengths	Vulnerabilities
Coping	Solves problems effectively and independently at times Seeks help and uses it at times	Unable to solve problems without considerable assistance Disintegrates under pressure Unable to marshal personal resources in time of crises Becomes immobilised or defeated under challenge Lacks resiliency Difficulty adapting Finds it hard to deal with crises, transitions and real, imagined, or anticipated losses
Treatability	Participates in programmes and treatment likely to be of benefit at times Cooperative at times Wants to succeed at times Responds well to biological and social treatment	Perceives no point in attempting change Unengaged at times Uncooperative at times When more or less obliged to participate in programmes, merely "goes through the motions"

of the risk and the need to plan longer term is less suitable for a CARM formulation. Here, a SMART care plan goal can be linked to Steve's SLF. It was agreed to develop Steve's narrative Static-Dynamic Risk Formulation (see Table 10.4) into a Static-Dynamic Formulation Care Plan (see Appendix 4 for a template).

In completing this particular care plan, it is important to clarify what dynamic stable factors were present at the time of the index offence and whether these are present now. Factors not currently present are marked as crossed through in the START. In terms of acute dynamic factors those present in the past are recorded and monitored as to whether they re-emerge. The nature of Steve's static factors indicates that progress is likely to be slow. Indeed, this care plan is intended to be long term. It is also quite broad in terms of interventions. Each of these may be further usefully planned using the SMART methodology described earlier. Developing a therapeutic relationship with Steve was of key importance here in being able to as accurately as possible to identify potential past factors. Sometimes, however, this is not possible and here the team must resort to examining notes and police reports. Using the plan over the course of 12 months, reductions were noted in the presence of two stable-dynamic factors: anger dyscontrol and poor coping strategies. It was subsequently possible to modify these in subsequent START reviews as occasional anger dyscontrol and erratic use of coping strategies.

Table 10.4 Steve's Static-Dynamic Risk Formulation and Care Plan – Physical Assault (with or without weapons)

Steve's Static-Dynamic Risk Formulation and Care Plan – Physical Assault (with or without weapons)		
Static factors	Dynamic stable factors	Dynamic acute factors
Young age of first offence: History of violent behaviour (theft with violence, assault) – pro-criminal associates and beliefs (member of a gang for many years) "You need to put them down before they get to you, and when they go down, you better make sure they stay down" Index offence (leading to a prison sentence): criminal damage and assault causing actual bodily harm Cautions for fighting with peers at school; shoplifting; truanting – drinking alcohol and taking drugs with peers Arrested for physically assaulting his wife, attacking family with furniture and assaulting police officers when under the influence of alcohol and drugs Paranoid personality traits on The Million Clinical Multiaxial Inventory (MCMII; Million, 1997). History of substance abuse – cannabis and alcohol from an early age, pro-substance use beliefs Diagnosis of paranoid schizophrenia with persistent persecutory beliefs: ex-wife is arranging for gangs to hurt him and his family; family are out to steal from him and harm him; the staff treat him unfairly and want him locked in the system. History of non-compliance with medication and poor engagement with services and treatment. Limited insight into mental health state and need to be detained	High conviction in paranoid belief that there are conversations between staff and past gang members to harm him Hears voices telling him that he and his family are in danger Receives messages from the radio and TV confirming the aforementioned Erratic medication compliance Impulsivity, low frustration tolerance and anger dyscontrol Poor coping strategies Carrying weapons	Increased time spent with pro-criminal and pro-substance use peers Socialising more often in the local pub Feeling paranoid that someone is out to harm him Struggling to manage his increased paranoia and frustration Availability of weapons **EWS-R:** Frequent visits to pubs – increased alcohol and cannabis use Poor compliance with medication Frequently hearing a voice telling him he is in danger – increased feelings of anger Intrusive thoughts "Put others down before they get you" Becoming very easily offended with angry glaring
Reduce actuarial estimates in light of treatment response Build on Steve's acknowledgement (during RGPI) of past offences and discourage minimisation Encourage need to recognise and manage own personal risk and relapse factors in the future	Work on developing emotional regulation skills Social skills work Building trust PBS plans to reduce verbal aggression and socially inappropriate behaviour	**Short-term risk management plans** Support Steve to use his coping strategies Behavioural interventions, TBCT for in-situation beliefs Staff monitoring of behaviour Staff monitoring and review of medication

Utilising Individual START Items for Care Planning Purposes

Here we have found two items from the START particularly helpful. Firstly, "Insight", which covers the extent to which the individual recognises and understands the necessity for managing early signs of relapse and risk. Secondly, "Treatability", which concerns the person's ability to engage with and benefit from social, biological and psychological interventions. The RRES (Meaden et al., 2012) is helpful here in being able to assess and monitor levels of engagement across three domains. For example does the person score primarily in the domain of agreeing with treatment and basic relationships or do they show evidence of more active participation? A lack of strength in these areas will likely mean that team efforts will have to focus on intervening when early signs are present, as well as adapting the social environment to better manage setting events. Interventions will also be needed at the reinforcement level utilising behavioural interventions based on differential reinforcement principles (see also Chapter 6). In Steve's case, both of these areas were highlighted as being especially problematic. For Steve, these were readily incorporated into the earlier levels of care planning as they were common problems across a number of situations. For other areas and other service users, other types of care planning may be better suited: SMART or CARM-informed PBS plans.

Case Study: Otis

Otis is a 45-year-old male who was transferred to his local CRU following multiple acute and A&E admissions. Otis is diagnosed with schizophrenia and has a long history of drug use. He is moreover diagnosed with ADHD. Otis used to live with his mother who is in her late eighties, but she could not take care of his needs and had to move into a care home. Otis's mother purchased a small flat for him to live in. His older brother died when Otis was 14, and later his father died when he was 25. Otis has struggled to come to terms with their deaths ever since.

Otis struggles with ADL and his flat was found to be in a very unkempt state. He was not taking his medication regularly and had become paranoid that someone would attack him at home. He frequently heard people moving around in his flat or knocking on the door though it seemed that no one was there. He was also a regular cannabis user and would take drugs and drink alcohol to manage his paranoia, believing that it helped him to feel calm. However, when he drank alcohol, this would make him feel low in mood and he would start to experience suicidal ideation and thoughts of not wanting to live anymore. This would lead Otis to take overdoses, and he would either present to A&E or he would call the police or his mum to let her know what he had done so she could get help for him. When the overdoses were further explored, Otis explained that he would drink as it helped him to feel calm and to help with feelings of sadness associated with thinking about his family and how alone he believed he was. Otis admitted this would further lower his mood and he would become suicidal, having thoughts of wanting to join his brother and father.

Due to his poor medication adherence, self-neglect, substance use and repeated admissions to the ward following overdoses, Otis was referred to the CRU to support him with his difficulties. Once there, Otis continued to leave his room in an unkempt state. He struggled with washing and dressing. It was also noticed that Otis would sleep in the day and drink a lot of coke and coffee in the evening, he would request both zopiclone (which was already prescribed) and lorazepam to help him sleep. When the staff questioned him about the lorazepam, Otis would become irritable and demanded they give him the tablet as "*I need it to help me sleep*". Should the tablets not be forthcoming, Otis would start to hit himself on his arm with his fist; some staff would give him the lorazepam to stop this behaviour whilst other staff would explain this is not the best way to deal with sleep difficulties. Otis reported that he was being treated "unfairly" as he believed the staff members were deliberately withholding his medication because they wanted to punish him. In those instances, Otis would stop and retreat back to his room and throw items around, he would pull objects and posters off the wall or throw items around the corridor or in his room whilst swearing at the staff, calling them "racist bigots".

For Otis, it was readily apparent to the team that the key risks presented concerned substance use and attempted suicide risk. Here, we illustrate those aspects of our SAFE formulation and care planning most relevant to address these related risks. These were evident from the narrative static-dynamic risk formulation completed during the START process:

> Otis lives alone and has limited social contact. He spends much of his time in bed or on the settee ruminating about the past. He sleeps poorly, drinks and smokes cannabis to cope with his low mood. Around anniversaries and other significant events (linked to his brother and father) his substance use increases. At these times he becomes suicidal and has

> *thoughts of wanting to join his brother and father. Otis will go out to the shops and visit several to collect paracetamol and buy alcohol. Back in his flat he continues to drink which lowers his mood further. He will subsequently take an overdose, Otis will then panic and call for help.*

1   Otis's GPRI

Main Goals:

(a) To live in supported accommodation
(b) To be free of being haunted by the past.

Key Barriers Agreed From the RGPI

(a) Dependence on substances and prescribed medication to manage his emotions
(b) Poor sleep.

It emerged during the interview that Otis had at several points been offered counselling and therapy to talk about his complex bereavement, but he had frequently failed to follow through on these.

2   Otis's START (see Table 10.5)

These areas of the START were agreed by the team as being those most implicated in Otis's suicidal behaviour. Otis agreed to meet with the unit psychologist and OT with whom he got on well. Initially, meetings focused on how Otis was finding his time on the unit and completing the RGPI to build rapport and trust. Subsequently, relevant START areas were shared with Otis and it was put to him that as he always reached out for help, he did not really want to die but that he struggled to cope at times. It was agreed that one way forward would be to complete a care plan together.

Since being admitted to the unit, this behaviour had not been demonstrated and so time was taken to sensitively review past incidents with Otis. The pattern was always the same (as per the previous narrative risk formulation). However, Otis still struggled to manage his emotions and experienced paranoid thoughts on a daily basis which needed to be carefully considered in implementing any intervention plan to both build trust and prevent a further relapse. This process is captured in Table 10.6.

After completing the plan, it was shared with the MDT and Otis and his mother, who expressed a lot of concern about him and continued to be involved in his care. It was decided to devise three specific care plans to work on.

Table 10.5 Otis's Key and Critical Area Items for Substance Use and Suicide

START areas	Strengths	Vulnerabilities
Emotional state	Good spirits at times Sense of humour Ability to experience emotions Mood appropriate to circumstances at times	Pessimistic at times Emotionally withdrawn Lethargic Feelings of worthlessness at times Hopelessness Irritable Angry Emotionally restricted Adverse effects on self or others when under influence
Substance use		Uses illegal substances Indiscriminate intake Denies need for treatment (if indicated) Use is out of control Intoxicated Dependent
Social support		Non-availability of social support Inadequate social network
Insight	Makes connections between thought and action Applies facts to own state and circumstances Acknowledges mental disorder and the need for interventions	Does not identify and/or manage personal risk factors No recognition of early signs of relapse
Coping	Seeks help and uses it	Unable to solve problems without considerable assistance Disintegrates under pressure Unable to marshal personal resources in time of crises Becomes immobilised or defeated under challenge at times Lacks resiliency at times Difficulty adapting Finds it hard to deal with crises, transitions and real, imagined or anticipated losses Unengaged at times Uncooperative at times
Treatability		

Table 10.6 Otis's Static-Dynamic Risk Formulation and Care Plan

Otis's Static-Dynamic Risk Formulation and Care Plan for Suicidal Behaviour (taking overdoses)		
Static factors	Dynamic stable factors	Dynamic acute factors
Death of both brother and father Past overdose attempts (reported five past overdose attempts – include both over-the-counter and psychiatric medication) Diagnosis of paranoid schizophrenia and depression History of substance misuse	Living alone in his flat – subjective loneliness Poor concordance with medication Reports of not grieving for the loss of both brother and dad Paranoid beliefs that others do not care for him Poor coping skills Mum in care home and not being able to see her much Interpersonal relationship difficulties Low mood Poor sleep	Increase in paranoid ideation and social isolation Anniversaries of brother's and father's death Increase in drinking to help alleviate low mood Access to over-the-counter tablets Increase in suicidal ideation **EWS-R** Increase in sleep difficulties Resumes drugs and alcohol abuse Non-compliance with medication Not engaging with services and other people Not answering the phone or answering the door Room looking unkempt Poor hygiene and self-neglect
Reduce actuarial estimates in light of treatment response Build on Otis's acknowledgement (during RGPI) that he does not want to end his life Support the need to recognise and manage own personal risk and relapse factors in the future	Help him to build therapeutic and social relationships – engaging in groups and activities Work on emotional regulation TBCT to address paranoid beliefs Enhance coping strategies and social skills Substance abuse work Promote access to bereavement counselling	For staff to give Otis space to talk about how he is feeling and promote sleep hygiene Increase supervision and monitoring/team visits when in the community for signs of substance use or hoarding of medication and other pills For staff to encourage Otis to use his coping strategies

Table 10.7 Otis's SMART Goal for Developing a Social Network

Otis's SMART goals

Spending time with others	When?	Who?	Achieved?/ Comments
I want to have a supportive network of friends and others			
Play draughts or dominoes two times each week	By June 2019	Healthcare assistant	Achieved *Coloured Green*
Play draughts or dominoes two times each week	By August 2019	Healthcare assistant and a service user	Achieved *Coloured Green*
Play draughts or dominoes two times each week	By September 2019	Service user	Achieved *Coloured Green*
Join the weekly cooking class to cook some Afro-Caribbean food	By October 2019	OT	Achieved *Coloured Green*

3   Building Relationships and Social Support: SMART Care Plan

Otis reported that he felt "alone" and that no one truly cared for him. He had a small number of relationships on the ward and appeared very close with his named nurse. It was felt it would be helpful for Otis to build therapeutic alliances with other members of the team and peers as an initial step, so that he was not reliant on only one particular person. A SMART Goal Plan was developed (see Table 10.7) which included different staff engaging in activities that Otis enjoyed such as playing draughts and dominoes, attending activities with peers such as movie groups, joining cooking classes and playing in the weekly pool tournament. Also, this offered the opportunity to help him to build social networks that he might find supportive. In the longer-term, the aim was for Otis to visit his local cultural centre which offered a range of activities and social support.

In a related care plan, Otis was encouraged to practise social skills training (Bellack et al., 2004). This was to enable effective interactions with others and to be able to maintain supportive relationships.

1   Engaging in Recreational Activities

Whilst not part of Otis's static-dynamic risk formulation narrative, the OT raised concerns amongst the team that Otis was very sedentary and tended to take part in only solo activities. Building on SMART goal 1, it was agreed to support Otis to engage in other activities. A Quality-of-Life Card Sort was used to identify further interests Otis might like to engage in and to help him to develop new hobbies and activities for both himself and others. This intervention would help him further to develop relationships and hopefully sustain them. These interventions would need to be regularly reviewed and adjusted if difficulties arose. Otis identified that he would like to go to the cinema again (with other peers) and join a specialist Afro-Caribbean cookery course.

2   Emotional State and Bereavement Issues

These were long-standing problems for Otis. A member of the team was allocated to spend time with Otis once a day to encourage him to talk about how was feeling. The team could then help him to explore any worries or persecutory beliefs he had about the staff, with staff being open and honest about what they were thinking and why they did what they did (TBCT). This helped to build therapeutic relationships, improve Otis's awareness of others' internal world (including their motivations) whilst also gently offering alternative non-persecutory explanations for why the staff were acting in the way they were.

Otis also agreed to meet with the unit psychologist to work on developing his coping strategies to support his EWS-R plan. These sessions involved work on substance using the Cognitive-Behavioural Integrated Treatment (C-BIT) approach (Graham et al., 2004) and developing emotional regulation skills (relaxation and self-soothing exercises). Locally, a bereavement support group was identified and Otis agreed to attend this with support.

Using these care plans over the next six months, Otis gradually engaged more and more with other peers on the unit and had signed up to a cookery course. He had been on two trips out to the local cinema and developed a good relationship with two other peers. He had also attended two meetings at the local bereavement support group. He found this very difficult but was encouraged by how welcome he had been made to feel and had been able to use some of his coping strategies to manage his distress afterwards.

Summary

This chapter demonstrates how the different SAFE formulations can be used to devise several types of care plan. All have the shared goal of reducing barriers and enabling recovery. Care plan interventions are based on a shared understanding of the service user's unique inner world, allowing a clear identification of treatment targets based on their life and recovery goals in an effort to increase social participation. Reformulation of difficulties using new information can then be used to refine and update these care plans, supporting new or existing service user goals. Regular reviews of the impact of care plans through the routine use of our templates, the START and RRES can enhance the planning of care by assessing the effectiveness of the interventions (see Chapter 12). This grounds the care provided in a psychologically informed and systematically evaluated, service user-focussed approach to recovery.

Chapter 11

Applying SAFE to Other Settings

In developing SAFE, we have been clear that our focus has been on those with complex mental health and behavioural needs who are hard to reach and treat. Service users with these presentations most commonly receive care in specialty rehabilitation and forensic services. However, they will also require periods of acute care and are increasingly to be found under the care of generic Community Mental Health Teams (CMHTs) with the erosion of specialist mental health services in some areas (Edwards et al., 2022). There are significant challenges in providing SAFE in these setting due to short lengths of stay and/or reduced staffing ratios. In this chapter we describe how we have adapted the SAFE approach for use in these settings.

Community Mental Health Teams

Within our local CMHTs, more than 25% of the population have received a diagnosis of some form of psychosis. Whilst a proportion may present with complex behavioural needs, they may fail to meet the threshold for specialist services or there may be significant waiting lists for these services. A recent report by the Kings Fund (Gilburt, 2018, p. 12) concluded:

> NHS mental health trusts are struggling to staff existing services on a day-to-day basis and, while actions to implement routine safe staffing levels are evolving, the lack of available staff, particularly nursing staff, at a national level continues to undermine this.

Singh (2000) highlighted a number of barriers to the effectiveness of CMHTs:

1   Lack of a clear and targeted responses to care
2   Inadequate resourcing
3   A backlog of continuing care cases
4   Staff members who are reluctant to take on those who are difficult to engage
5   Increased demands from primary care
6   Difficulty keeping up with advances in evidence-based treatments

DOI: 10.4324/9781003082811-12

7   Varied key working practices
8   Poor communication between services
9   Staff burnout.

"Inadequate resources, especially the rapid reduction in acute bed numbers and pressures of bureaucracy, excessive and poorly managed workloads and the blame-culture have all made community working stressful, and in some cases ineffective" (Singh, 2000, p. 417). Twenty one years on, many of the observations made by Singh (2000) remain relevant today. CMHTs currently remain under-resourced with high staff turnover and remaining staff members managing higher caseloads than ever. As such, the remaining staff have even less opportunity to hold their service users in their mind as they work through the list of tasks and priorities. Regular line management and clinical supervision may be pushed back in order to meet service demands. Alongside new ways of working due to COVID-19, this means that more staff members are working in isolation and remotely, further limiting communication across other MDT professionals and services. MDT meetings are typically focused on how to address the service users' current presenting problems, meaning repeated revisiting of the same service user as the team try to address one problem at a time but struggle to address the source of the problem that may be maintaining their difficulties. This could be due to lack of time to formulate the difficulties and/or not having the available resources to address root causes. Hard-to-reach complex service users often present in crisis multiple times and may disengage from treatment and their risk left unmonitored.

Using SAFE in a CMHT

In amongst all these stressors, Singh (2000) suggested a number of interventions to improve the effectiveness of CMHT working, including having effective leadership, regular team workshops and shared learning, team risk assessments and prioritising and responding to individual cases. The SAFE approach offers possible solutions to addressing some of these problems. Useful starting points are the START to properly assess risk as a team with a recovery focus and our SLF, which can serve as a useful review tool highlighting those that appear stuck in the system, recognising where there is progress (to instil hope) and indicating where referral to another service may be helpful. It can also identify cases where problem behaviours are creating a significant barrier to recovery and thus can be prioritised for further work.

Case Study: Richard

Richard is a 44-year-old male diagnosed with paranoid schizophrenia. He has a long history of paranoia since his early teens. He reports that he hears a female voice scream and a male voice laughing and whispering at him, almost constantly.

Richard's parents separated when he was young and his mother remarried. He recalls problematic behaviour at school and was diagnosed as having Oppositional Defiant Disorder. Richard reported that his stepfather physically abused him and Richard ran away from home aged 13. He went to live with his father until his early twenties. He said he had an "on and off" relationship with his father and at one point he physically assaulted him whilst also hitting, kicking and breaking the walls, doors and furniture in the house. Richard reported that he did not know why he did this and showed remorse for his behaviour. He said he tried to have contact with his mum, but felt he could not trust her and he could not forgive her for not supporting him when he was being assaulted by her partner. Richard described having flashbacks and nightmares of his stepfather's abuse.

Richard has been under the care of a CMHT for over ten years. He engages poorly, frequently misses appointments and denies having any mental health problems. Richard has a significant history of violence. Growing up, Richard said he "fell in with the wrong crowd". He started to hang around with people who were older than him and engaged in illegal activities such as criminal damage and vandalism. Richard explained that he felt like he was part of a family. Richard had several incidences of stealing cars and joyriding with his friends and destroying the cars afterwards. During one of these incidences, Richard sustained a head injury and was taken to hospital, where he was kept for a couple of days.

Richard has been arrested for several physical assaults. As a teenager he punched his girlfriend in the face, and she sustained a fractured jaw, for which he was found guilty of assault occasioning actual bodily harm. Richard was given a conditional discharge and a fine. Richard was also arrested for common assault following an incident where he threw a pint glass that hit a barmaid. When drunk, Richard has been known to approach customers at ATMs and demand money off them; if they do not comply, he has physically assaulted them. Richard has also been involved in gang-related violence, attacking several members of different gangs over the years.

Richard has a good relationship with his father. Richard has two children from a previous relationship and sees them every fortnight in the presence of his father. He says his children make him feel happy.

Richard appears to experience paranoid ideation, describing an incident in which he threw an object at a person who he felt was laughing at him. Looking back, Richard now believes the person was laughing with others and not actually at him. Richard moreover has some paranoid beliefs about his neighbours. He believed that they placed devices on the ceiling and they were listening to his conversation. One night after several days of drinking, he banged on the neighbour's door, shouting at them, telling them to come out and threatening to assault them with a knife for spying on him. The neighbours called the police. Richard was assessed by the mental health team and referred to an acute ward where he was diagnosed with paranoid schizophrenia and started on medication. Richard reports that he still hears voices and does not like to go outside as he worried that if someone looks at him in the wrong way, he will become angry and attack them. He continues to have nightmares and flashbacks of his stepfather hurting him and having past fist-fights.

While on the caseload of the CMHT, Richard started to hide himself away and not go out without someone being with him. He continued to experience voices as well as nightmares and flashbacks. The psychiatrist referred Richard for a psychological assessment for flashbacks and nightmares and anxiety management. Richard attended the assessment session, reporting that he felt better for talking and agreed to be seen for a trial of therapy. Richard attended therapy but disengaged after five sessions as he struggled to talk about his past convictions as part of his assessment.

Information From Richard's SAFE Process

As Richard disengaged with the psychological therapy services, it was felt that he needed a team approach to understand his presentation and needs (especially his risk) as he had been in the service for many years and had not obviously progressed much. As Richard struggled to talk about his past convictions, it was difficult to complete any standard risk tools with him; neither would he engage in completing a RGPI. It proved extremely difficult to engage other members of the team to collaborate in work with Richard.

Following a discussion about Richard's case with the MDT, it was agreed that the team would benefit from gaining a shared understanding of Richard, his presenting problem, his past and current risk behaviours and how best the CMHT can support him and to identify if his needs could be best met elsewhere.

It was decided that a START would be the most helpful place to assess Richard's risk behaviours, while an MDT shared formulation was used to make sense of where his difficulties (both psychological and behavioural) may have originated from and what was keeping them going. The electronic care record was reviewed to inform the START and also devise a developmental timeline for Richard. A Case Formulation Team was assembled including the psychologist, psychiatrist, nurse prescriber and the team manager. One hour per week was set aside over five weeks to develop this work.

Richard's START: Key Strengths and Vulnerabilities

To help prioritise which areas to start with, START THREAT (Threats of Harm that are Real, Enactable, Acute and Targeted) items were reviewed. This is especially important in CMHTs where the team's ability to closely monitor and quickly respond are limited due to the community nature of the service and the lower staffing ratios when compared to inpatient care, forensic services and AOTs. For Richard, violence (verbal and physical aggression) had been present in the review period, so this was prioritised for immediate assessment and formulation in order to inform care planning. In addition, a second opinion was requested from forensic services to explore whether he may benefit from a more specialist team.

For Richard, several vulnerabilities were identified that were deemed as likely to be critical items and could be linked to Richard's narrative static-dynamic risk formulation. In Richard's case, there are two possible routes to physical assault:

1. Richard has underlying antisocial attitudes, viewing violence as a solution to conflict in relationships. He has problems with anger control and this is significantly exacerbated by alcohol use, which he uses to manage his nightmares, panic attacks and flashbacks. Lack of money for alcohol can be a triggering event.
2. Stopping medication increases Richard's paranoia and his male voice tells him to hit others (ego-syntonic and in keeping with his own attitudes) if he is slighted in any way (others perceived to be laughing at him or staring at him). He is more likely to comply when disinhibited due to the effects of alcohol.

Richard's Vulnerabilities as Identified as Likely to Be Critical Items on the START

1. Relationships
2. Mental state
3. Emotional state
4. Substance use
5. Impulse control
6. External triggers
7. Attitudes
8. Medicine adherence
9. Conduct
10. Insight
11. Coping
12. Treatability

Richard adamantly refused to look at his substance use and it was felt that supporting him to develop and utilise coping strategies might prove more productive. It was also proposed that as some incidences were related more to antisocial attitudes permissive of criminal behaviour, the initial focus would be on those factors associated with assaultive behaviour due to a relapse in his mental health. For this reason, it was also decided not to work at this point on his command hallucinations as these were ego-syntonic in nature. After careful review it was agreed to try to address three broad areas. Consideration was also given to not only which barriers were the most significant but also to those which may best respond to intervention.

1   Poor engagement with services and non-compliance with medication
2   Mental state – EWS-R and EWS-P, paranoid ideation
3   Coping strategies

Interventions for Richard

As Richard had already disengaged with psychology input due to increased levels of paranoia, it was felt that as a starting point, the team would focus on helping him to engage more with services. A key question for informing the development of interventions for Richard was how does the CMHT team address risk behaviour when Richard attends only scheduled appointments erratically for medication review and does not have any other contact with services? How could Richard be engaged and/or motivated to develop skill to manage his own behaviour in the community?

Richard was allocated two care coordinators to increase monitoring opportunities. These were experienced care coordinators who worked to build a relationship with Richard. A small case team was assembled who were the key point of contact for Richard, in order to increase the number of familiar faces for him and in an effort to manage the impact of paranoia and anxiety. This was used to build a stable relationship with Richard and encourage him to develop care plans that he was involved in writing. As the relationship developed the Case Formulation Team were able to develop a combined EWS-R and EWS-P plan for Richard in the form of a safety plan (see Table 11.1), in keeping with our focus on behaviour. Here, the emphasis is on keeping the service user and others safe and well. It helpfully moves away from the notion of relapse and by implication "illness" models and begins a shared dialogue concerning problem behaviours as the key factor in preventing recovery. As part of this process, the team psychologist supported the CFT to develop a coping repertoire with Richard.

Given the high levels of risk highlighted by the START, more regular reviews with the psychiatrist were scheduled, alongside regular monitoring visits from the case team. It was agreed that the EWS-R plan would be used by Richard's psychiatrist at these more regular reviews.

Following the care plan Richard has not had a further admission for over two years and has had no further incidents of assault.

Table 11.1 Richard's Team-Based Safety Plan

Possible Triggers		
Drinking alcohol everyday all day	Problems with benefits and lacking money	Changing care coordinator

Early Signs and Ways of Staying Safe and Well	
What do I and what others notice?	*What I and the team can do to help?*
Early: Having more frequent nightmares and panic attacks Feeling anxious – experiencing pins and needles and heart racing Scanning the environment for sources of threat Experiencing racing thoughts	**Me:** Practise self-calming and self-soothing strategies Go out for a walk in nature (local park) **Team:** Offer to take Richard out for a coffee Check if Richard is having any benefit or money problems Practise a relaxation strategy with him
Middle: Experiencing intense flashbacks Frequent panic attacks Becoming paranoid and angry	**Me:** Practise self-calming and self-soothing strategies Go out for a walk in nature (local park) Keep busy with my daily routine Try and ignore other people when I think they are having a go or staring at me Walk away **Team:** Offer extra medication Practise a relaxation strategy with him Go over coping strategies and gently explore and challenge any paranoid ideas (using TBCT techniques)
Late: Becoming quite paranoid Hearing male voice telling me to do stupid things: punch him in the face Avoiding going out – staying in drinking all day	**Me:** Ask for help and more frequent visits Stop drinking and take my meds **Team:** Increase visits – review drinking and medication compliance Take him out for a walk and a coffee

Using SAFE in a Home Treatment Team

A Home Treatment Team (HTT) aim to provide rapid assessment and crisis management and enable service users to be treated outside of hospital as far as possible and remain in their usual place of residence (Burns et al., 2001). They aim to facilitate more rapid discharge from an acute setting, offering respite to carers from the demands of caring and to provide timely and accessible help to persons experiencing psychiatric and psychosocial crisis (Crisis Resolution Home Treatment Operational Policy, 2007). The team mainly consist of psychologists, nurses and psychiatrists.

The staff face a number of similar difficulties to CMHTs; especially in terms of staffing. The National Audit Office (2007), Healthcare Commission (2008), Mind (2011) and the Centre for Social Justice (2011) questioned the effectiveness of these teams in meeting service users' needs. Carpenter et al. (2013) undertook a systematic review of crisis teams, including an analysis of patient's feedback of their experiences of HTT services. They found that 85% were satisfied with the care they received and 92% said they would use the service again. However, some service users reported that due to resource issues, they had experienced a lack of frequent and prompt communication which caused them anxiety and stress. A particular challenge is the need to maintain relationships when shift patterns mean that several different people will usually be visiting each service user. Some service users found such inconsistency difficult, particularly if staff were inadequately briefed and did not work well together as a team. Lyons et al. (2009) reported that some service users complained that teams focused too much on prescribing and dispensing medication and too little on practical and emotional support.

SAFE is precisely designed to improve communication through the use of shared formulation, thus enabling all of those involved in the person's care to understand particular difficulties and have a consistent approach to delivering quality care. It seems clear that service users require a HTT when they are in crisis, when their behaviour becomes of concern to themselves and/or others. Using a structured risk assessment such as START may be too time-consuming for a HTT as they hold a large caseload and the nature of the work often means that most of the team will be out in the community and may not have the opportunity to come together to look at one service user with such depth. Time under the care of these teams is also short. CARM formulations can be particularly helpful here as they can be completed in a single session (such as a case bust) and can be built on (e.g. with an EWS-R plan) to support other community teams who are involved in the ongoing care of the person.

Case Study: Emma

Emma is a 36-year-old female diagnosed with schizophrenia. She has been under the care of her local CMHT on and off for a number of years. She has a history of disengaging with mental health services and being non-compliant with medication often leading to being discharged.

Emma is a devout catholic. When she was nine years old, she was molested by her older cousin who was aged 14. Emma believed that she had encouraged the abuse and that God was punishing her for

it. For many years Emma wore loose-fitting clothes. She prayed frequently to God seeking forgiveness. Emma said she could never tell
her parents what had happened as they would never believe her. When
Emma was going through puberty she struggled with the changes and
boys at her school would make comments about her. It was around
age 14 that Emma started to hear a voice saying that she was "dirty", a
"slag" and "unclean" and to "strip off". She assumed the voice was the
devil. This frightened Emma as she felt she had further drifted away
from God. Emma recalls that her prayers to God increased and she
started to engage in fasting to cleanse herself of her sins and subsequently started to lose weight. She also showered more frequently and
rubbed her skin in the shower until it was red and sore. When going to
school Emma became low in mood and spent a lot of time in bed. Also,
she stopped washing and dressing. This concerned the family and she
was referred by the GP to her local CMHT where she was diagnosed
with schizophrenia. Emma was prescribed antipsychotic medication
and her voices lessened and her mood and appetite improved.

Emma managed to complete college and went to university where
she started a relationship. However, she found out that her partner
had cheated on her and after ending the relationship Emma found out
that she was pregnant. Emma knew she could not keep the baby as
her parents would be extremely angry at her for finding herself in this
position. She also worried about terminating the pregnancy as this was
against her religion. Emma soon heard the voice come back, saying
that she was "dirty", a "slag" and "worthless". Emma became increasingly desperate and drank a bottle of bleach alongside an overdose of
several boxes of paracetamol and codeine. She was rushed to hospital
and when Emma came around, she was extremely disappointed that
she had not ended her life nor the baby's life. Emma continued to
hear both male and female voices laughing at her. Emma was referred
to a psychiatric ward and was treated with antipsychotics. Her family
supported her with the pregnancy, but it was agreed that she would
give the baby up for adoption. Emma returned back to her family and
started a part-time job at a supermarket. Emma continued to attend
church and seek forgiveness for the baby she felt she had abandoned.
She found solace in the church, and she slowly stopped engaging with
mental health services and weaned herself off medication.

At age 30 Emma got married. Unfortunately, Emma experienced
domestic abuse in this relationship. The voice of the devil returned
as well as the laughter and the sounds of a baby crying. Emma started

to not shower and was praying, asking God for forgiveness. Emma would not wear much clothing as she would listen to the voice telling her to strip. Emma again tried to take another overdose, but her husband discovered her and called the ambulance. At hospital, Emma was dishevelled, obeying the voice's commands to strip off her clothes and screaming about hearing babies crying. Emma was referred to an acute psychiatric unit where she stayed for two months. During this time Emma was started on a depot.

Emma separated from her husband and moved back in with her parents. She saw herself as a failure and blamed herself for the problems in her life. She decided to go back to studying. Unfortunately, Emma struggled to concentrate and with the demands of the course subsequently stopped attending. During this period, she missed some of her depot injections also. The voices re-emerged and she started to believe that her parents worked for the devil and wanted to kill her. Emma stopped coming out of her room, she would not eat, wash or dress. Her parents became concerned and contacted HTT. Emma heard her parents make this call and she decided enough was enough and decided to end her life. She took another large overdose. She was again hospitalised and shortly transferred to the psychiatric ward. She was recommenced on depot and referred for psychological assessment on the ward.

Emma's CARM Formulation Process

As Emma had repeatedly taken overdoses over the years and having accessed a number of services, it was agreed at the HTT daily team meeting that it would be helpful to understand the overdose behaviour in more depth with the aim of preventing future crises. It was evident from Emma's presentation and her parent's accounts that there was a predictable pattern and set of behaviours that preceded these attempted suicides. Completing a stand-alone CARM formulation was agreed as this was becoming such a frequent behaviour. A CFT was assembled, including the community psychiatrist, HTT psychiatrist, community psychiatric nurse and psychologist. Emma and her family were also involved in the discussions. Using information gathered from her notes the team were able to complete a CARM template which was subsequently shared with Emma and her parents, (see Figure 11.1). During the meeting it was also agreed that she would benefit from an EWS-R plan so that Emma, the team and her parents can monitor her early warning signs of risk to more effectively mobilise help if needed. A risk formulation was also developed with input from Emma, her parents and the CFT for use by Emma, her family and services (see Table 11.2).

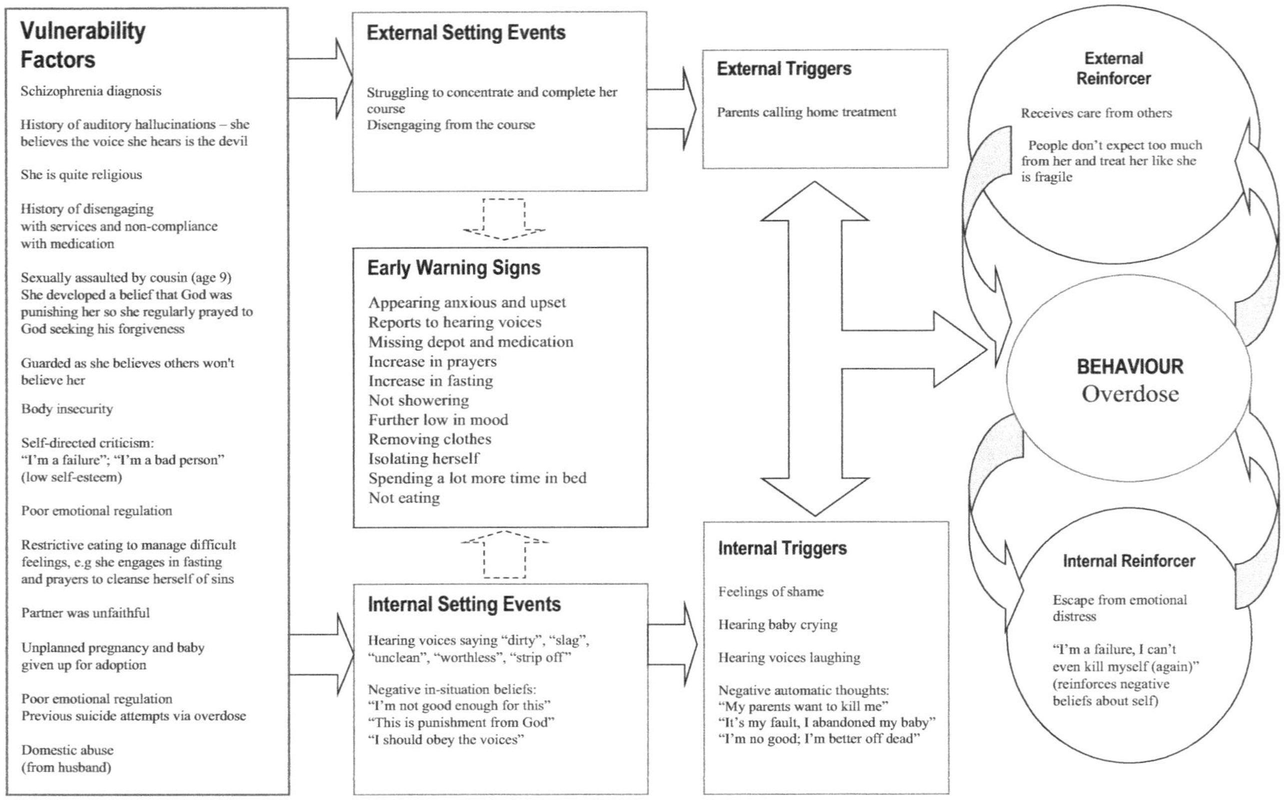

External Reinforcer

Receives care from others

People don't expect too much from her and treat her like she is fragile

BEHAVIOUR

Overdose

Internal Reinforcer

Escape from emotional distress

"I'm a failure, I can't even kill myself (again)" (reinforces negative beliefs about self)

External Triggers

Parents calling home treatment

Internal Triggers

Feelings of shame

Hearing baby crying

Hearing voices laughing

Negative automatic thoughts:
"My parents want to kill me"
"It's my fault, I abandoned my baby"
"I'm no good; I'm better off dead"

External Setting Events

Struggling to concentrate and complete her course

Disengaging from the course

Early Warning Signs

Appearing anxious and upset

Reports to hearing voices

Missing depot and medication

Increase in prayers

Increase in fasting

Not showering

Further low in mood

Removing clothes

Isolating herself

Spending a lot more time in bed

Not eating

Internal Setting Events

Hearing voices saying "dirty", "slag", "unclean", "worthless", "strip off"

Negative in-situation beliefs:
"I'm not good enough for this"
"This is punishment from God"
"I should obey the voices"

Vulnerability Factors

Schizophrenia diagnosis

History of auditory hallucinations – she believes the voice she hears is the devil

She is quite religious

History of disengaging with services and non-compliance with medication

Sexually assaulted by cousin (age 9)
She developed a belief that God was punishing her so she regularly prayed to God seeking his forgiveness

Guarded as she believes others won't believe her

Body insecurity

Self-directed criticism:
"I'm a failure"; "I'm a bad person" (low self-esteem)

Poor emotional regulation

Restrictive eating to manage difficult feelings, e.g she engages in fasting and prayers to cleanse herself of sins

Partner was unfaithful

Unplanned pregnancy and baby given up for adoption

Poor emotional regulation
Previous suicide attempts via overdose

Domestic abuse
(from husband)

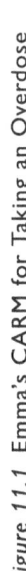

Figure 11.1 Emma's CARM for Taking an Overdose

Table 11.2 Emma's EWS-R Plan for Taking Overdoses

Target behaviour: Overdosing

Signs client may show before engaging in this behaviour (Type of EWS-R)	How the client normally behaves (Typical presentation)	How client behaves when unwell (Atypical presentation)	Action: What to do to help the client (Interventions)
Breakdown in relationship; struggles to complete something important e.g., course work etc (Contextual sign)	Emma is a quiet, shy and reserved person. She is usually able to complete tasks in her day-to-day life.	Emma can appear upset and overtly anxious. She may start to make comments such as "it's my fault"; "I'm not good enough" and become easily frustrated	Emma to speak to a friend, or someone she trusts to get a balanced perspective on any given situation which has upset her
Hears voices- "dirty", "slag" "unclean "and "worthless" and the voice tells her "strip off" .	When Emma is stable, she hears the voices, but not so frequently and these are almost at a whisper level and she can distract herself from them	She starts to become distracted by voices and is upset and tearful and may start to remove items of clothing (which we suspect is an attempt to stop the voices)	Using coping techniques that help her feel calm, such as "square breathing". Tell herself she is okay Remind Emma that an increase in intensity and frequency of voices is indicator that she is stressed and she would benefit from managing her stress (rather than trying to appease the voices). Write down Negative automatic thoughts and when calm try to generate alternative explanations Remind Emma that her response is a reaction to bad and upsetting news, but this is temporary and support is at hand and she does not have to listen to the voices (it has not helped before). Ensure there is no excess medication or tablets in her house and if there are to remove them Request appointment with CPN and possible medical review

Early stages

(Continued)

Table 11.2 (Continued)

	Signs client may show before engaging in this behaviour (Type of EWS-R)	How the client normally behaves (Typical presentation)	How client behaves when unwell (Atypical presentation)	Action: What to do to help the client (Interventions)
Middle stages	Stop taking medication (Visual sign)	When stable and life is going well, Emma will be concordant with her mediation	Emma starts to miss her medication and stops collecting her repeat prescriptions from the GP.	For parents to call in and let mental health services know that they suspect Emma is relapsing. Services to contact GP to see if she is regularly picking up her medication. Mental health services to make contact with Emma and if needs be to arrange a home visit and medication review.
	Increase in praying Increase in fasting (Visual signs)	Emma attends Church every Sunday and observes prayers and fasts	There seems to be a change in her presentation, i.e. not going out, isolating herself, missing her parents phone calls Emma becomes preoccupied with prayers as a way to seek solace, comfort and seek forgiveness. This means that her daily routine can become disrupted and she can miss her medication, hospital and CMHT appointments	Family to check in on Emma and if they notice increase in prayers remind her that this is may be a sign that she is feeling more stressed. Remind Emma that she is not a bad person and to spend time with her engaged in a valued activity (such as stitching, knitting, walking etc). Call mental health services and request a home visit and medication review To signpost to spiritual care or to a priest she trusts to support Emma with her increased prayers and to provide spiritual education around this.
	Not showering Low in mood (Visual signs)	Emma would wash and shower at least 4 times a week minimum	Emma stops showering, stops brushing her teeth and hair and wears the same clothes and does	Parents to prompt Emma to wash and dress and reward her with activities she likes. Request an urgent home visit from CPN. To help Emma engage in structured activities and for family and friends to go out with Emma out for a walk To contact Home Treatment and to request a medical review

(Continued)

Table 11.2 (Continued)

Signs client may show before engaging in this behaviour (Type of EWS-R)	How the client normally behaves (Typical presentation)	How client behaves when unwell (Atypical presentation)	Action: What to do to help the client (Interventions)
Removing clothes (Visual sign)	Emma dresses modestly and does not remove items of clothing	Emma starts to wear minimal clothing and sometimes no clothes. She appears very down and tearful. Again Emma maybe listening to the voices commands to "strip off".	To contact Home Treatment and to request a medical review
Isolating herself more (Visual sign)	Emma is a friendly person and has friends in the church and mental health service.	Stops all contact with outside world	For any signs of late stage EWS-R, please action the following: To arrange urgent medication review
Spending a lot of time in bed (Visual sign)	She is usually active throughout the day	She becomes very insular and lost in listening to the voices and becomes increasingly distressed Thoughts of being not good enough increase in frequency and increase the chances of taking an overdose	Call HTT and to discuss the possibility of hospitalisation
Not eating (Visual sign)	Emma usually eats 3 meals a day but is not a 'big eater'	Emma starts to lose weight and refusing food at time and not wanting to eat.	

Late stages

Intervention

An EWS-R plan was devised with Emma and her parents. Also, it was agreed that when Emma returned to the care of the CMHT, then longer-term intervention could be attempted focused on her beliefs and past trauma.

Emma did not engage with the team psychologist but over the next two years she did not need a further period under the HTT or need any acute hospital admission. She did have one further crisis, but with timely intervention this was managed effectively by the CMHT.

Summary

In this chapter we have explored the use of the SAFE approach in other settings. Whilst there may not always be the team infrastructure to undertake larger assessments and formulations like the START, we have demonstrated that other shorter formulations of CARM and EWS-R can be completed as stand-alone formulations and care plans.

It is important throughout this to work within any MDT that other services are involved in the process and to have care continuity with person's recovery with a consistent care coordinator assigned to the service user. SAFE formulations can then promote this continuity of care. This facilitates a person-centred and needs-adapted approach and is more likely to enable recovery. Moreover, using the SAFE approach in this way can reduce repetition and over assessment and achieve a clearer understanding of service user's needs.

Chapter 12

Measuring Outcomes and Capturing Change

Introduction

Of key importance throughout the SAFE approach is that it is evidence-based and flexible, being able to meet the complex needs of service users, one of the cornerstones of the need-adapted treatment approach (Alanen, 1997). It is therefore of critical importance that we assess needs and monitor the effects of our efforts. Monitoring outcomes and capturing change is a routine aspect of SAFE. In this chapter we describe some of the ways in which we have been monitoring progress in services where we have implemented the SAFE approach.

Importance of Practice-Based Evidence

It is recognised that alongside traditional and well-established approaches to gathering evidence of the efficacy of interventions, such as through randomised controlled trials (RCT) and meta-analysis, there is increasingly a place for "practice-based evidence" (Green et al., 2008). One of the challenges in applying evidence from the research literature into practice is the ecological validity of the research, particularly in the representation of service user populations. The population that is the focus of SAFE is, by definition, hard to reach, as evidenced in several studies (e.g. Cowan et al., 2012; Meaden et al., 2014). This group are not typically well represented in RCTs or other research of psychological interventions that require regular attendance at repeat appointments. There remains therefore a need to evaluate current practice, including the consideration of whether new interventions might be meaningfully adapted, evidenced (practice-based evidence) and incorporated for this hard-to-reach group.

Meaningful Outcomes

In keeping with an increased emphasis on recovery (e.g. Slade et al., 2014), outcome needs to be tailored and meaningful to the individual. One of our core aims within the SAFE framework is to enable individuals and teams to effectively manage distressing emotions and challenging behaviours. Our layered approach to

DOI: 10.4324/9781003082811-13

shared formulation is at the heart of this, with an emphasis on identifying the idiosyncratic and personally specific maintenance factors that are related to the formulation question (e.g. what behaviour, what barrier) and linking these to specific meaningful outcomes.

Whilst focusing much of our attention on problem behaviours and barriers when conceptualising an outcome, we believe that there is a need to move beyond these to consider well-being and quality of life as part of living a life worth living (Papadopoulos et al., 2013). This may include consideration of individual factors as guided by shared assessment and formulation, such as measurement of beliefs (e.g. Beliefs About Voices Questionnaire; Chadwick et al., 2000), cognitive processing (e.g. The Awareness of Social Inference Test; McDonald, 2012) or symptoms (e.g. Calgary Depression Scale; Addington et al., 1993). Furthermore, outcome assessment should be sensitive to what may be objectively small yet subjectively significant aspects of well-being. These should be relevant to achieving fuller social participation and leading a personally meaningful life. These outcomes are not the easy bedfellows of RCTs, but they are key to engaging and working collaboratively with those who may be struggling with their relationship with services and the interventions they offer. Given these considerations, it should be apparent that there is a need to be somewhat creative in our evaluation of SAFE practice.

An important consideration is to ensure that measurement of outcomes does not become an onerous and burdensome task for those delivering the service. Ideally, it should also not be seen as detached from the clinical process. Evaluation of outcome must capture what is being routinely achieved, enabling care teams to gain a sense of purpose, retain hope and enabling all members to routinely capture change and adapt interventions accordingly to changing needs. We therefore advocate that the measurement of change should become as much a part of routine practice as care planning. In other words, it becomes embedded within services and thus allows a more dynamic consideration of progress that can be linked to care planning (i.e. are the care plans working?) as well as aiding service-related planning and (at least in the UK) commissioning (i.e. is the service working?).

Routine Assessment of Clinically Meaningful Factors

It is imperative that services are clear about their aims as this will guide the choice of assessment (see Chapter 2). Enhancing engagement and managing challenging behaviours has been discussed as key when working with service users with complex psychosis and behavioural needs (Meaden et al., 2014) and as such, measurement of these domains can provide useful information at a service and individual level. We would add to this the measurement of activity and functional behaviour, often referred to as "activities of daily living" (ADL), as there is evidence that ADLs are impaired in people with psychosis and that this and the functional outcome are closely associated with cognitive deficits (Fett et al., 2011; Velligan et al., 1997). With this in mind, we have established a small suite of measures that can be used routinely within services to monitor outcomes as part of care planning, known locally as the Rehabilitation Assessment Suite. These Clinician-Rated Outcome Measures (CROMs) assess service user engagement, problematic behaviour and functional activity in daily living and are designed to be completed as an MDT, though they can be completed individually if needed (e.g. by a key worker who knows the service user well). Items on the measures and associated scoring scales are designed to be defined behaviourally to aid accurate assessment and scoring in the team. This moreover encourages the service to focus on things that can be changed (e.g. Leff et al., 2002) such as behaviours rather than those that may be less amenable to change, such as symptoms.

The RRES (Meaden et al., 2012) can be used to assess how well a service user engages with the rehabilitation process. The scale contains 16 items regarding compliance with medication (1 item), agreement with treatment and basic relationships (5 items), active participation and openness (10 items). Items are measured on a 5-point scale ranging from "never relates well with the team" to "always relates well with the team". Higher scores indicate better engagement with rehabilitation.

The CBC-P (Meaden & Hacker, 2010) aims to classify problematic behaviour across two dimensions: the recency/frequency of the behaviour and the severity of the behaviour, using 11 subscales. This includes intentional/deliberate harm to self, verbal aggression, physical aggression against objects, physical aggression towards others, sexually inappropriate behaviours, fire risk behaviour, compulsive behaviour, acquisitive behaviours, absconding, socially inappropriate behaviours and behavioural deficits.

The assessment uses two sets of rating scales. Items are firstly rated in terms of recency/frequency of occurrence on a scale of "0" (Never present) to "8" (has occurred in the last week). If an item attains a higher rating than "0" on the recency/frequency scale, it is subsequently rated in terms of severity of the specific behaviour (when it occurred) on a scale of "0" (no challenge) to "4" (direct and imminent harm to self or others).

The Resettlement Scale (see Appendix 6) is completed to assess clients' functioning across eight areas: basic self-care, basic living, social interaction, community, financial, self-management of mental health, physical health and recovery. These items are rated on a 5-point scale (from "No Ability" to "Independent"). The results can of course inform care planning but can also be used to consider the appropriate level of support that the service user will benefit from upon discharge.

We suggest that these measures are completed initially on entry into the service (e.g. within the first two months) and then routinely every three to six months (depending on mean length of stay) to align with the care plan review process. Scores can be compared longitudinally to track progress and map change. With this in mind, we have recommended the use of a standardised report in our rehabilitation services completed by members of the MDT across each of the three assessment domains (i.e. engagement, ADLs, challenging behaviour). Rather than having headings split by discipline (e.g. separate sections for nursing, psychology and occupational therapy feedback), disciplines are encouraged to contribute to the same functional assessment sections for a written consideration and discussion of service user progress across the three domains. The current scores obtained in the measures are plotted against the historical scores to facilitate visual comparison and track progress. In line with the core principles of the SAFE approach, the use of this report to structure care planning reviews every three to six months allows for an integrated consideration and discussion of progress within the team, with the service user, family and others involved in their care. Plans can then be developed based on these systematic and structured considerations ready to be reviewed through the assessments at the next care plan review meeting.

Using Assessment to Guide Care Planning

It is helpful to have a structured system to link assessment with service aims, service user goals and care plans, and we have previously used GAST to support this (Meaden & Hacker, 2010). A fundamental but often overlooked aspect of the care planning process is the way in which assessment feeds back into the modification of care plans. Plans showing little change will need to be reviewed. We should ask at this point:

1 What else can be tried?
2 Have we exhausted all of the possible intervention options?
3 Is it time to move on to other possible goals (e.g. is this as good as it gets for this goal currently)?

At one of our units, we have had the benefit of working particularly closely with multidisciplinary colleagues. Here has been developed an effective and clear system of monitoring care plan outcomes between assessment periods. We locate this at the end of our care review document (i.e. after the assessments and interpretations), and it serves to link the findings from the assessments discussed in the previous section to care plan goals. An example of how this may look is replicated in Table 12.1 and provides an example of how the SAFE process can be linked to care plan goals and reviews.[1] Once again, RAG (i.e. Red, Amber, Green) ratings help with clarity: goals that have been achieved are highlighted in a green font, those partially achieved are highlighted with an amber font and those not yet started are indicated with a red font.

From Table 12.1 we can see that the service user, Andrew, has contributed to the overall long-term goal in each domain, which is located next to the standardised headings (e.g. "Community Integration: I want to be able to live safely in the community and stay out of hospital"). These headings are used to capture the services' broad care plan aims; however, they are devised with service user input. Under each heading are the care plan goals associated with that domain, alongside identification of who is responsible, by when this is to be achieved and what progress

Table 12.1 Linking Assessment Recommendations to Care Plan Monitoring

SMART goals/recommendations	When?	Who?	Achieved?/Comments
Medication management and staying healthy: I would like to be able to manage my medication on my own		**When?**	**Achieved?/Comments**
Andrew to move to level 3 of the self-medication programme	June 2021	Andrew and named nurse	Partial – Andrew requires occasional prompts to attend
Community integration: I want to be able to live safely in the community and stay out of hospital		**Who?**	**Achieved?/Comments**
Andrew to practise his road safety with the OT on Unit shadowing his trips	May 2021	Andrew and OT	Achieved
Andrew to practise making his own way to the local shops to buy his 1:1 cooking ingredients and return	June 2021	Andrew	Not yet achieved
My general support needs: for everyone I work with to have a better understanding of my mental health needs and how best to manage these		**Who?**	**Achieved?/Comments**
Andrew to develop "staying well plan" to reduce relapse risk	May 2021	Andrew and Psychology	Achieved
Andrew to attend regular mindfulness drop-in sessions to develop coping skills for mental health needs	May 2021	Andrew and Psychology	Partial – has been attending (with a prompt) but not yet completed take-home practice
Andrew to reduce the number of cigarettes he smokes by following the plan designed with named nurse	June 2021	Andrew, named nurse and MDT	Achieved

	When?	Who?	Achieved?/Comments
My life skills and interests: I would like to be able to look after myself independently in the community			
Andrew to complete 1:1 cooking once a week with support from staff	May 2021	Andrew and MDT	Achieved
Andrew to practise new recipe following guide developed for him by OT	June 2021	Andrew and OT	Not yet achieved
Andrew to complete budget skills training with named nurse	June 2021	Andrew and named nurse	Ongoing
	When?	Who?	Achieved?/Comments
Discharge planning: to leave rehabilitation and to live in the community as independently as possible			
To complete Joint Commissioning Tool ready for submission to panel to assess funding required for support package	June 2021	OT, named nurse and psychology	Partial – awaiting outcome from cognitive assessment

has so far been made. These areas can be considered, reviewed and updated at regular care planning meetings, and additional items can be added as needed. As a common pattern within our SAFE approach, RAG ratings help to clearly identify whether (and why) goals have been achieved or not. This offers a concise way of monitoring and reviewing progress within services.

Using the SLF as an Outcome Tool

A familiar observation from discussion with staff teams is a growing recognition that important changes for our service users are not always readily open to capture by established psychometrics. Even the measures discussed in this volume such as the RRES and CBC-P at times fail to fully capture the subtle shifts and changes in the lifeworld of our service users. We have noticed that it is often the less obvious changes that seem to be the most meaningful and personally significant for staff, service users and their families, and these may be lost in a rush to measure that which can be captured as part of routine outcome evaluation.

Case Illustration: Jocelyn

Jocelyn has received a diagnosis of schizophrenia and been in an inpatient rehabilitation unit for the last 18 months. She spends most of her days in her room, usually getting out of bed after noon, requiring numerous prompts and reminders from staff to attend to her physical healthcare. She demonstrates flat affect and rarely initiates conversations. The staff report that there has been little change during her time in the service. In team supervision sessions, the staff have described how they believe that they have "let her down" and feel caught between the need to move Jocelyn on (due to "bed blocking") and the desire to "do more" for her.

However, Jocelyn's family report that they are pleased with the changes they have noticed. They explain how she will now send them a text every week on her phone (albeit briefly) and occasionally contribute to family discussions on a shared social media account. She has also been telling her mother about her trips out of the unit once a week with the occupational therapist. Family members report that they had not been aware of this interest in family and unit life prior to the inpatient admission, and this gives them hope for Jocelyn and her recovery.

Considering such difficulties in fully capturing meaningful aspects of the service user's lifeworld, we have been advocating the use of more qualitative and descriptive outcome evaluation. To this end, we have been trialling the use of the SLF (Meaden & Hacker, 2010) to capture change. This formulation tool was originally designed to help focus the service and team on key areas that may act as barriers to service user recovery, linking recovery to personally meaningful social roles and activity. As we have completed reformulations with this tool, we have been struck by changes in the form and presentation of symptoms, internal and external barriers to participation. We now advocate the routine use of service reformulations to highlight areas of improvement and deterioration. In Table 12.2 we can see an example reformulated SLF for Jocelyn. Identified barriers to recovery that are judged to have improved are highlighted in green (indicated in Table 12.2 as G), barriers that have become worse are highlighted in red (indicated in Table 12.2 as R), while continued improvements over more than one SLF are highlighted in blue. This colour coding quickly emphasises how observed strengths, needs and barriers are seldom ever static.

This simple process offers a powerful way of capturing areas of change, and such changes can be listed and described in reviews and reports to evidence progress. In Table 12.2 we see that there were some key areas of change for Jocelyn, and these can be used to have an open discussion in the team about the steps forward for her. The green items indicate that there were some areas of activity that held meaningful purpose for Jocelyn; however, unit staffing issues and the recent recognition of her road safety needs were areas that required additional attention. It was agreed that weekly trips out to visit her family could be planned with Jocelyn and incorporated into road-safety training at the unit so that she could develop her skills in accessing the community. This was also used as motivation to help her to get up on those days and to manage her self-care more effectively.

The SLF tool can be used routinely by services to monitor changes in social engagement and recovery. The simple structure allows for clear and yet individually tailored tracking of recovery progress. Items rated as green can be taken to care reviews to highlight progress and ensure effective interventions continue, whilst items rated as red can be reviewed and appropriate care plans be developed. However, as a broad tool designed to capture the range of idiosyncratic factors associated with recovery, the SLF can struggle to identify particular areas that need to be prioritised. As such, we also advocate using the START tool in a similar manner to provide a structure designed to identify specific factors relevant to capturing and understanding changes in risk and treatment response.

Use of the START as an Outcome Tool

As discussed in Chapter 4, we advocate the use of SPJ tools to inform the SAFE processes. In particular, we find the use of the START (Webster et al., 2004) to be a useful way of capturing dynamic risk and treatability factors that can be used to develop shared risk formulations and management plans. In addition to this, we have also used the START to monitor and capture outcomes – as the detailed structure and familiar anchor points for rating items offer various ways to conceptualise change. Here, we describe two approaches to using START data to monitor progress: identifying change at the individual level to guide specific care planning processes (similar to the SLF process already discussed) and identifying patterns or commonalities at a service level.

Table 12.2 Jocelyn's Service Level Reformulation Changes

Service Level Formulation

Service User Name   Jocelyn

Date Completed

SU Identifier (information system number)

SLF Version 2

Symptoms and impairments	**External barriers**
What ongoing symptoms (including diagnosis where relevant) impairments and disabilities the person has as a result of their diagnoses? Diagnosis: schizophrenia Flat affect Low motivation (but pleasure remains intact, as reports enjoying trips out) **G** Limited self-initiation of activity Ideas of reference: believes the radio is talking about her	*What restrictions and barriers are placed upon the individual externally/from others?* Lack of hope in the care team regarding recovery No clear discharge pathway identified Requires escort off Unit due to road safety risks **R**
Internal barriers	**Participation/Personal recovery**
What does the person do themselves that creates barriers for their recovery? Requires multiple prompts to attend to personal hygiene Stays in bed until late morning/afternoon Difficulty following complex instructions (e.g. cooking) Unable to cross the road safely **R** Requires multiple prompts to engage in activities Does not initiate contact with others Now initiates contact with family **G** Limited social activity/interest in social activities but will now contribute to family discussions on social media group **G** Reports that enjoys trips out with OT **G**	*What does the person want to participate in but is limited due to symptoms, impairments and barriers?* Unable to return back to live with her mother due to self-care needs Personal hygiene and low activity motivation limits access to local community Unable to go for walks in community due to need for escort

Using the START to Capture Individual Change

The routine completion of the START offers the opportunity to compare previous scores over time for a given individual and review whether any change has occurred either at the factor level or the individual item level. At the supporting item level, changes are identified by crossing items out that are now absent and colouring these as red (indicated in this chapter by R) for deterioration and green (G) for improvement. At the individual dynamic factor level when a score has been increased then, similarly, this can be highlighted as green for an area of improvement and red for an area of deterioration. Lastly, if an item is rated as a key item (i.e. strength), then it is coloured green; where it is a critical item (i.e. vulnerability), then it is coloured red. Critical items can then be used to inform EWS-R plans (see Chapter 5).

An example of the dynamic factors section of a START completed in this way can be seen in Table 12.3, while in Table 12.4 the supporting information for the dynamic factors (where change has been observed) is replicated. This illustrates how, in this individual's case, social skills have been observed to improve; the increase in score from 0 (no evidence of strength) to 1 (partial evidence of strength) is supported by endorsement of items highlighted in green (e.g. joins in group activities, initiates conversations). Modifiers can be used to clarify areas, such as "feels **some** satisfaction in social situations" is "**mostly** pleasant and polite" or "lacks manners **at times**", with the improvement again highlighted in green. This method allows us to track quite subtle changes over time so that they can be used to inform care planning and also highlights to the team, the individual and their carers what has changed. This latter function is particularly important in helping the team to perceive change in service users where change can be slow and idiosyncratic and therefore helps to maintain the team's hope for recovery. Changes can be highlighted and taken to care reviews for planning purposes but also used by the clinical team to understand changes in the service user's risks and response to intervention. During team formulation and reflective practice sessions, we carefully but consistently highlight these changes thereby endorsing the appropriateness of ongoing care efforts.

Items from the START can also be easily summarised and collated to take for discussion in care reviews. This can involve summarising the number of strengths and vulnerabilities that have shown improvement/deterioration and using the supporting item information to offer a description of the changes. Experience suggests that such a clear grounding in team-based evidence (including, where possible, service user accounts and descriptions) can be useful in focussing the efforts of the team on shared care plan goals. Furthermore, sharing areas of improvement with service users can enhance motivation and engagement in rehabilitation.

Using the START to Understand Services[2]

One additional benefit to routinely completing the START is that we can use the data to examine specific cohorts of service users, including change over time. We find the START is well suited to this approach as summaries can be developed across various dimensions of measurement including the severity scales for the various behavioural categories (e.g. verbal aggression, suicide) and the strength and vulnerability scores for the 20 dynamic factors.

We have been involved in assessment of local rehabilitation services and we provide some data here as an example that was collected as part of routine service evaluation (Simpson, 2019). In this evaluation, the START was routinely used as part of the SAFE approach within a long-term high-dependency inpatient service.

Table 12.3 Changes in START Areas

Key item	Strengths			START items	Vulner- abilities			Critical item
	2	1	0		0	1	2	
G	○	G	○	Social skills	○	●	○	○
○	○	○	●	Relationships	●	○	○	○
○	○	○	●	Occupation	○	○	○	○
G	G	○	○	Recreation	●	○	○	○
○	○	○	○	Self-care	○	G	○	R
○	○	○	●	Mental state	○	○	●	○
○	○	●	○	Emotional state	○	○	○	○
○	●	○	○	Substance use	○	R	○	○
○	○	○	●	Impulse control	○	G	○	R
○	○	○	●	External triggers	○	●	○	○
○	○	●	○	Social support	○	●	○	○
○	●	○	○	Material resources	●	○	○	○
○	○	●	○	Attitudes	●	○	○	○
○	○	●	○	Medicine adherence	○	●	○	R
○	●	○	○	Rule adherence	●	○	○	○
○	○	●	○	Conduct	●	○	○	○
○	○	○	●	Insight	○	○	●	○
G	○	G	○	Plans	●	○	○	○
○	○	○	●	Coping	○	●	○	○
○	○	●	○	Treatability	○	●	○	○

Originally printed in, and reprinted here with the kind permission of, Webster, C. D., Martin, M., Brink, J., Nicholls, T. L., & Middleton, C. (2004). *Short-term assessment of risk and treatability (START)*. St. Josephs Healthcare, Hamilton and British Columbia Mental Health and Addiction Services.

The most recent START data available in the service was used to obtain a "snapshot" of the needs of the service users. This is a particularly poorly understood group, only being formally recognised quite recently (Joint Commissioning Panel for Mental Health, 2016). We summarise the data here to illustrate the type of information that can be derived from routine use of measures such as the START.

Demographics

Data representing a total of 26 service users were included in the evaluation. The mean age was 54.13 years old. The mean number of years since first admission to mental health services was 29.46 years. Diagnoses included paranoid schizophrenia (84.62%), schizo-affective disorder (11.54%) and bipolar disorder (3.84%). About 73% were detained under Section 3 of the Mental Health Act, 15.39% were detained under Section 37 and 11.53% were detained under Section 37/41. The ethnicity of the service users included Afro/Black-Caribbean (34.62%), White British (30.76%), Indian (19.22%), African (3.85%), Bangladeshi (3.85%), Black British (3.85%) and White and Asian (3.85%).

Table 12.4 Changes in START Item-Rating Supporting Evidence

START items	Strengths	Vulnerabilities

Social skills	Pleasant
	Polite
	Joins in group activities **G**
	Initiates conversations **G**
	Good communication skills
	Socially appropriate
	  behaviour
	Feels some (**G**) satisfaction
	  in social situations
		Avoids many social situations
		Isolated/Withdrawn/Shy
		Loner
		Difficult to engage
		Lacks manners
		Does not communicate well
		Immature
		Intrusive

Recreation	Aware of recreational
	  opportunities
	Uses leisure time
	  constructively
	Enjoys recreational
	  activities **G**
	Plans activities for self and
	  others **G**
	Willing to be helped to
	  develop interests and
	  hobbies **G**
	Takes regular physical
	  exercise
		Largely sedentary
		Does not want to engage in
		  recreational pursuits
		Refuses to participate in new
		  activities and pro-social
		  projects
		Has few if any hobbies or
		  interests
		Does not undertake regular
		  physical exercise

Self-care	Carries out basic personal
	  hygiene with some
	  prompts **G**
	Maintains personal space
	  in satisfactory condition
	  with some prompts **G**
	Appropriately dressed
	Normal sleep patterns
	Normal eating patterns
	Accepts health teaching
		Personal hygiene is maintained at
		  less than minimal levels only **G**
		Personal space is disordered and
		  unclean **G**
		Dresses in idiosyncratic or
		  inappropriate fashion
		Does not follow health teaching
		  (diabetes)
		Abnormal sleep patterns
		Abnormal eating patterns
		Abnormal fluid intake

Impulse control	Restrained Calm Contained Deliberate Controlled Thinks before acting Considers consequences Tolerates frustration	Overwrought Erratic Out-of-control Excited **R** Risk-taking Impulsive **R** Acts on spur of moment Does not anticipate consequences Poor frustration tolerance

Plans	Socially acceptable
	Realistic **G**
	Focused
	Future-oriented
	Goal-directed **G**
	Has plans to achieve short-
	  and long-term goals
		Goals are absent or vague
		Unrealistic
		Unacceptable
		Has neither short-term plans nor
		  long-term goals

Understanding Risk and Challenging Behaviour

Using the START risk incident scales, the number of cases recorded as having ever demonstrated key risk or challenging behaviours as identified by the START was calculated (i.e. static risk). Violence (96.15% of the sample) and self-neglect (84.62% of the sample) were the most frequently observed historical risks in this cohort sample.

The number of service users exhibiting challenging or risk behaviours in the four months prior to the most recent START was also collated (i.e. dynamic risk). This suggested that self-neglect was the most frequent (84.62% of the sample), followed by verbal aggression (73.08% of the sample). It is also interesting to note that service users who were vulnerable to victimisation were the third most frequent (42.31% of the sample showed recent evidence of this).

The mean severity of the observed risk behaviours as rated by the START was explored. These scales range from 0 to 4 (except for the sexually inappropriate scale, which ranges from 0 to 3) with higher scores indicating greater severity. Mean scores in the sample were calculated by summing the observed scores and dividing by the number of service users recorded as having demonstrated that behaviour. This indicated that when verbal aggression occurred, it was, on average, at a level towards the higher end of the severity scale, past the mid-point (mean = 2.84; standard deviation = 1.01). The next highest severity behaviour was physical aggression against objects (mean = 2.33; standard deviation = 1.12) and the third highest was self-neglect (mean = 2.09; standard deviation = 0.87).

Also, we examined the mean vulnerability and strength factor scores (which range between 0 and 2 on the START). These factors are found to contribute to the presence or absence of risk or challenging behaviours and are routinely incorporated into SAFE formulations we have described previously in this volume. Lack of social support (mean = 1.65; standard deviation = 0.63), poor insight (mean = 1.50; standard deviation = 0.71) and deficits in social skills (mean = 1.46; standard deviation = 0.51) were observed to be some of the most critical areas of vulnerability for this sample. Limited substance misuse (mean = 1.50; standard deviation = 0.71), access to material resources such as adequate finances (mean = 1.42; standard deviation = 0.64) and minimal external triggers (mean = 1.27; standard deviation = 0.78) were observed to be key areas of strength for this cohort.

From this, we can see that it is possible to use routine assessments to derive summaries of the services within which SAFE is implemented. Reviewing such data sets at regular time intervals then allows the monitoring of service-level outcomes over time. For example by using the data derived from routine assessment we have been able to focus efforts on developing our understanding of self-neglectful behaviours and how to work with these, offering training to support staff teams working with these needs. Also, it ensures that these behaviours are themselves not neglected as they are often obscured by the focus on more immediately "high risk" behaviours such as physical aggression. Similarly, it is interesting to observe that the top three areas of observed strengths identified in the recent service evaluation (Simpson, 2019) were all externally driven (limited access to substances of abuse, access to resources and external triggers), indicating the perceived importance of social factors (i.e. CARM external factors, see Chapter 9) in the management of risk and discharge planning within inpatient rehabilitation services. Such data can be used to guide service-related changes, such as targeting training for staff teams on areas of identified need – for example in social skills training (one of the highest rated service user vulnerability factors in the recent service evaluation).

Summary

This chapter has described a variety of ways to measure outcome and capture change for our service users when using the SAFE approach. This has included the use of standardised psychometric tools developed for use in this population (e.g. the RRES and CBC-P) alongside more qualitative methods that harness the idiographic power of formulation (e.g. the SLF). In particular, we have illustrated the benefits of using the START tool to monitor changes at the service user and organisational level. Future work can explore the effectiveness of these approaches and refine their use to ensure that SAFE remains rooted in evidence-based principles and practice.

Notes

1 Special thanks to Hannah Lake, Senior Occupational Therapist, for her ideas and work in this section.
2 Many thanks to Jonathan Simpson for his contributions to the data discussed in this section.

Concluding Remarks

SAFE offers a structure to guide and inform MDTs in their work with some of the most complex mental health and behavioural needs. The formulations used as part of this approach have been developed to meet the functions typically required within recovery and rehabilitation services. In the preceding chapters we have described the use of these to guide the development of a shared understanding of service user needs to enhance effective collaborative teamwork. We have attempted to articulate a way of working with teams and service users that offers hope and opportunity for innovation – particularly for times when feeling stuck or unsure of how best to proceed. Distress and problematic behaviour associated with psychosis (both within the service user and the team) are the focus of understanding and intervention, and it is our belief that it is this clarity that enhances the utility of SAFE.

In Chapter 2, we outlined our process for identifying where and under what circumstances SAFE may be best introduced. Of course, not all teams and services will be receptive to the notion of SAFE. This can be particularly prevalent in services that are dominated by a culture where traditional psychiatric practice and "silo" ways of working between professional groups are firmly established. We understand that wider service pressures, preferred models, service history and team personalities also play a role in the decision to adopt new ways of working. Nevertheless, we feel strongly that going along with the status quo will not add meaningfully to the care process for the needs we have described here. Under these circumstances, we may usefully consider team-based Long-Term Supportive Psychotherapy as an alternative option (Meaden & Hewson, 2015).

For SAFE to be most effective, there needs to be open and clear communication between team members, alongside clear guidance and support for the approach from senior leadership. In the short term, implementation of SAFE is likely to be resource-intensive and as such it requires a strategic level of agreement to ensure consistent implementation – change in a system requires a sustained level of energy for it to become "the new normal". We have found that where SAFE has appeared to work best is where there have been several MDT members who have worked to consistently guide and implement the approach within the team. Identifying local "champions" of the approach drawn from the MDT and supporting

DOI: 10.4324/9781003082811-14

them through training and supervision can be one way of improving the delivery of the approach. Such team members can be useful in holding in mind that where SAFE can been consistently implemented, it offers an opportunity to develop and enhance the care of service users, grounded in thorough and robust assessment and formulation processes. In other words, it is an approach that facilitates the work of the team rather than necessarily adding to it.

Rigid and unthinking reliance on general guidelines may also be a problematic aspect of healthcare services that can stifle innovation and change. This can result in an organisational tendency to support a tickbox approach, advocating the prescription of interventions such as individual CBT-P or family therapy without an adequate understanding of the context to the evidence base and associated limitations. In such situations, it can be useful to review the function of services and consider the use of data collected as part of routine outcomes (such as that described in Chapter 12). This can facilitate an exploration of the effectiveness of interventions derived from general guidelines contrasted with those derived from an understanding of the particular needs and difficulties of the people using the service (as advocated in SAFE).

There are limits to all interventions, and SAFE will not address all problems. It was developed as a way of working with service users whose needs are associated primarily with difficulties with distressing psychosis. This focus is one of the strengths of SAFE, with the process of deriving an understanding of the difficulties and developing associated interventions informed from the evidence base of this particular area. Other areas of need that are less closely linked with psychotic difficulties may be less amenable to the use of SAFE; however, we have started to make an attempt to apply some of the principles of SAFE in other settings (Chapter 11). These will require further research and evaluation to evaluate their utility in such settings.

In clinical cases where SAFE has been attempted but has not demonstrated effectiveness for meaningful recovery, we should be satisfied firstly that we have exhausted all available interventions and that we have fully assessed and measured progress. In these instances, the service user will at least have received a thorough assessment and formulation, and such information may be useful for them and their team in future, if only to describe and capture some of what was known and understood up to that point in their recovery. This can be used for future work with services to help guide understanding and care.

Research and evaluation are key to innovation and development. We have described how we developed our use of SAFE across the contexts within which we work including through service evaluation and consideration of routine practice-based evidence. It has been vital to review our own psychological knowledge, remaining abreast of developments in the field, considering where these might usefully be incorporated to improve our work for the people who use our services. We have moreover described ways in which we are attempting to measure change as part of evaluating the effectiveness of SAFE, and here there is further work that can help us to better understand the different aspects of SAFE and where these can be usefully adapted to enhance care. We urge readers to take the ideas we have articulated here and explore the evaluation of these within their own services; it is through this process that care can be adapted to better meet the needs of the people who use our services.

Importantly, although SAFE is an approach grounded on psychological principles (such as formulation, cognitive and behavioural theory), it is not solely the preserve of psychologists. We hope that we have made it apparent that by working holistically, communicating clearly and with a shared vision, we can harness the benefits that come from the knowledge and perspectives within the team (and service user and family). We offer SAFE as one way of capturing this knowledge and these perspectives, linking them to psychological theory to understand difficulties and distress and using psychological formulation to inform ways of enhancing recovery.

Appendices

Service Level Formulation Template

Service Level Formulation

Service User Name   SU Identifier (*information system number*)
Date Completed   SLF Version (*1st formulation, 2nd, 3rd etc.*)

Symptoms and impairments	External barriers
What ongoing symptoms (including diagnosis where relevant) impairments and disabilities the person has as a result of their diagnoses?	What restrictions and barriers are placed upon the individual externally/ from others?
Internal barriers	**Participation/Personal recovery**
What does the person do themselves that creates barriers for their recovery?	What does the person want to participate in but is limited due to symptoms, impairments and barriers?

Protective factors (*the service user's strength mitigators against relapse and risk*)

Three key recovery barriers (*potential care planning goals*)

1.

2.

3.

Guidance Notes

Impairments/Symptoms: looks at symptoms of the mental and physical well-being of a service user and how these could be preventing them from meeting their goals.

Internal barriers: refers to anything the service user does that may limit their recovery. It includes their attitudes and behaviours from their learnt life experience.

External barriers: are those that are outside of the service user's control that may limit their recovery, such as contact with friends and family and restrictions on leave.

Social participation: looks at meaningful social activities that the service user would like to do, however is unable to carry them out due to internal and external barriers that are preventing them from being able to meet their goals.

Protective factors: are those that mediate against risk behaviour and relapse, such as having prosocial friendships, engagement in meaningful activities.

Three key barriers: are the main barriers in preventing the person from meeting their goals and moving forward in their recovery. These can be used as part of their service user's care plan.

CARM Template for Active Behaviours

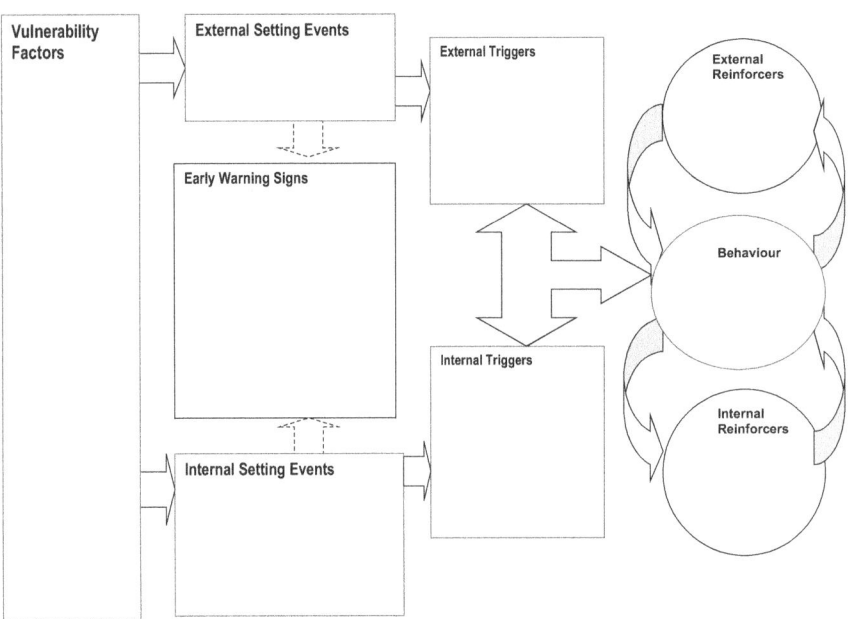

CARM Template for Passive Behaviours

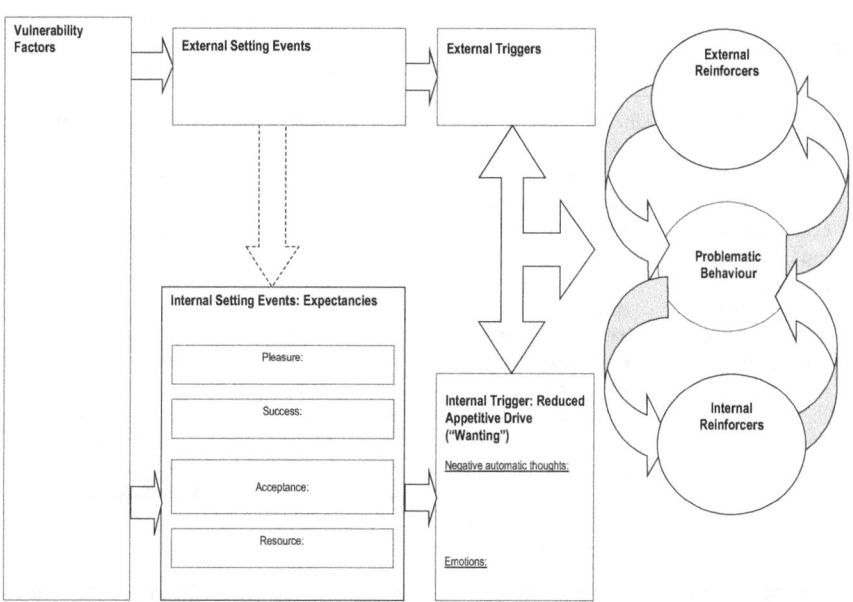

Static-Dynamic Risk Formulation and Care Plan

Target behaviour	Static factors	Dynamic stable factors	Dynamic acute factors
Operational definition (e.g. setting fire to own room, stabbing other inpatients with a knife, taking an overdose of prescribed medication)	Unchanging/ Historical in nature ♣**Demographic factors** (e.g. age, gender, number of offences) ♣**Idiosyncratic historical factors** (e.g. type of victim in previous assaults; lethality of methods in previous suicide attempts)	Factors responsible for driving the risk behaviour (the function of the behaviour) May change/ respond to treatment but slowly over time (e.g. trait anger; antisocial attitudes; chronic paranoid delusions; persistent depression, substance use)	Factors that most closely predict risk New or increases/ changes in stable dynamic factors (e.g. increased distress from voices; substance use conflict with partner) **Triggers? EWS-R&P?**
Care planning process CPA based upon structured clinical judgement using actuarial and other assessment tools as appropriate	**Prediction of long-term risk:** How likely is this person to repeat the behaviour compared to others? What is the nature of the risk posed and its likely impact/severity?	**Medium-long-term treatment targets** TBCT or individualised Development of social skills and coping strategies	**Short-term risk management plans** Support to use coping strategies; behavioural interventions, TBCT for in-situation beliefs

>>>>>>>>>>>>>>>>>*Each behaviour has its own risk trajectory* >>>>>>>>>>>>>>>>>>

>>>>>>>>>>>>>>> How factors interact to produce risk over time>>>>>>>>>>>>>>>.>>>>

Challenging Behaviour Record Sheet for Psychosis (CBRS-P)

Table A5 Challenging Behaviour Record Sheet for Psychosis (CBRS-P)

What was the behaviour?	Service user's EWS-R	Distant triggers	Immediate triggers	Intervention and effect? Reaction of others?	Service user's view?
Please describe the behaviour as accurately as possible	*What were the service user's presentation and behaviour like leading up to the event in the few hours or minutes before?*	*What events had occurred prior to the incident, which were not immediate triggers but may have contributed to making the behaviour more likely later on?*	What happened to make the behaviour occur at the particular moment that it did?	*What did staff do? What effect did this have? What did others do? What effect did this have?*	(When calm) What was the service user's views of what happened?

Resettlement Scale

Date Rated: Service/Unit:

Client's Name: Rater's Name:

To be completed with reference to clinical and psychiatric notes
For each item, please rate "*Level of Support Required*" on a scale of 1–5 (refer to the Rating Scale).

Please use the following rating scale to rate each individual item.

Level of support required
5 Carries out behaviour under own volition (i.e. independent)
4 Carries out behaviour only with prompting
3 Carries out behaviour only with assistance
2 Has the ability but does not carry out at all
1 No ability to carry out the behaviour/task

Basic self-care skills	Level of support required
1. Dresses appropriately	
2. Wears clean clothing	
3. Maintains personal cleanliness, washes when necessary	
4. Is appropriately concerned with grooming	
5. Maintains privacy when getting washed and dressed	

Basic self-care skills	Level of support required
6. Can prepare simple drinks and snacks	
7. Can prepare a basic meal	
8. Maintains appropriate standards of food hygiene	
9. Can safely use cooking appliances	
10. Can safely use dangerous objects	
11. Can safely use general domestic appliances	
12. Maintains acceptable levels of cleanliness	
13. Uses washing machine appropriately	
14. Hangs clothes to dry/uses drier	
15. Ensures a sufficient amount of sleep	
16. Is able to shop for food and other essential items	
17. Eats regularly and maintains an appropriate diet	
18. Has basic literacy skills to read instructions, correspondence, labels, signs	
19. Is able to use telephone for appropriate needs	

Social interaction skills	Level of support required
20. Can develop and maintain meaningful relationships with others	
21. Can maintain appropriate boundaries with others	
22. Can appropriately communicate their needs	
23. Has appropriate non-verbal skills	
24. Can be appropriately assertive	
25. Can resist exploitation from others	
26. Initiates and sustains a conversation with others	
27. Has appropriate family contact	

Community skills	Level of support required
28. Is able to access community facilities when needed	
29. Aware of personal safety and is "streetwise"	
30. Can navigate themselves around local community	
31. Is able to cross roads safely	
32. Is able to use public transport as needed	

Financial skills	Level of support required
33. Can budget for basic needs	
34. Pay bills when needed	
35. Shows evidence of knowing the worth of possessions/items	
36. Manages money transactions effectively	
37. Is able to recognise financial difficulty	

Self-management of mental health	Level of support required
38. Is able to develop and maintain a daily routine	
39. Is able to manage any ongoing negative symptoms effectively	
40. Is able to manage any ongoing positive symptoms effectively	
41. Able to employ effective coping strategies when needed	
42. Monitors for signs of relapse	
43. Is able to employ adaptive strategies for cognitive difficulties	
44. Seeks help appropriately	
45. Has constructive ways of managing emotional difficulties	
46. Is able to regulate substance misuse effectively	

Physical health	Level of support required
47. Can manage medication independently	
48. Is able to monitor side effects and seeks help when appropriate	
49. Attends check-ups (e.g. blood tests)	
50. Seeks medical advice when needed	

Recovery	Level of support required
51. Sets appropriate and realistic goals for the future	
52. Has identified aspirations	
53. Recognises own strengths and assets	
54. Is able to go about achieving goals in a systematic way	

References

Addington, D., Addington, J., & Maticka-Tyndale, E. (1993). Assessing depression in schizophrenia: The Calgary Depression Scale. *British Journal of Psychiatry, 163*(suppl. 22), 39–44.

Alanen, Y. O. (1997). *Schizophrenia: Its origins and need-adapted treatment.* Karnac Books.

Allen, D. (2020). *Positive behavioural support, what is it?* [video]. Retrieved March 29, 2020, from www.challengingbehaviour.org.uk/information/information-sheets-and-dvds/positive-behaviour-support.html

Allen, D., James, W., Evans, J., Hawkins, S., & Jenkins, R. (2005). Positive behavioural support: Definition, current status and future directions. *Tizard Learning Disability Review, 10*(2), 4–11.

Andreasen, N. C. (1982). Negative symptoms in schizophrenia: Definition and reliability. *Archives of General Psychiatry, 39*, 784–788.

Andrews, D. A., Bonta, J., & Hoge, R. D. (1990). Classification for effective rehabilitation: Rediscovering psychology. *Criminal Justice and Behavior, 17*, 19–52.

Andrews, D. A., Bonta, J., & Wormith, J. S. (2006). The recent past and near future of risk and/or need assessment. *Crime and Delinquency, 52*, 7–27.

Anthony, W. A. (1993). Recovery from mental illness: The guiding vision of the mental health service system in the 1990s. *Psychosocial Rehabilitation Journal, 16*(4), 11.

Appelbaum, P. S., Robbins, P. C., & Monahan, J. (2000). Violence and delusions: Data from the Macarthur violence risk assessment study. *American Journal of Psychiatry, 157*, 566–572.

Ayllon, T., & Azrin, N. H. (1965). The measurement and reinforcement of behavior of psychotics 1. *Journal of the Experimental Analysis of Behavior, 8*(6), 357–383.

Ayllon, T., & Azrin, N. H. (1968). *The token economy: A motivational system for therapy and rehabilitation.* Appleton-Century-Crofts.

Ballatt, J., & Campling, P. (2011). *Intelligent kindness: Reforming the culture of healthcare.* RCPsych Publications.

Beck, A. T., & Rector, N. A. (2005). Cognitive approaches to schizophrenia: Theory and therapy. *Annual Review of Clinical Psychology, 1*, 577–606.

Beck-Sander, A., Birchwood, M., & Chadwick, P. (1997). Acting on command hallucinations: A cognitive approach. *British Journal of Clinical Psychology, 36*(1), 139–148.

Beech, A. R., & Ward, T. (2004). The integration of aetiology and risk in sex offenders: A theoretical model. *Aggression and Violent Behaviour, 10*, 31–63.

Beer, B. (2006). Managing challenging behaviour. In G. Roberts, S. Davenport, F. Holloway, & T. Tattan (Eds.), *Enabling recovery: The principles and practice of rehabilitation psychiatry* (pp. 211–231). Gaskell.

Bellack, A. S., Mueser, K. T., Gingerich, S., & Agresta, J. (2004). *Social skills training for schizophrenia: A step-by-step guide*. Guilford Publications.

Bennett-Levy, J., Butler, G., Fennell, M., Hackman, A., Mueller, M., & Westbrook, D. (2004). *Oxford guide to behavioural experiments in cognitive therapy*. Oxford University Press.

Bennett, R., & Pearson, L. (2015). Group rational emotive behaviour therapy for paranoia. In A. Meaden & A. Fox (Eds.), *Innovations in psychosocial interventions for psychosis: Working with the hard to reach*. Routledge.

Benton, M. K., & Schroeder, H. E. (1990). Social skills training with schizophrenics: A meta-analytic evaluation. *Journal of Consulting and Clinical Psychology, 58*(6), 741.

Bernard, M., Jackson, C., & Birchwood, M. (2015). Cognitive behavioural therapy for emotional dysfunction following psychosis: The role of emotional (dys) regulation. In A. Meaden & A. Fox (Eds.), *Innovations in psychosocial interventions for psychosis: Working with the hard to reach*. Routledge.

Berry, K., Barrowclough, C., & Wearden, A. (2009). A pilot study investigating the use of psychological formulations to modify psychiatric staff perceptions of service users with psychosis. *Behavioural and Cognitive Psychotherapy, 37*(1), 39–48.

Berry, K., Haddock, G., Kellett, S., Roberts, C., Drake, R., & Barrowclough, C. (2015). Feasibility of award-based psychological intervention to improve staff and patient relationships in psychiatric rehabilitation settings. *British Journal of Clinical Psychology, 55*(3), 236–252.

Bieling, P. J., & Kuyken, W. (2003). Is cognitive case formulation science or science fiction? *Clinical Psychology-Science and Practice, 10*(1), 52–69.

Birchwood, M. (2015). Knitting up the ravelled sleeve of care: Sleep and psychosis. *Lancet Psychiatry, 2*(11), 950–951.

Birchwood, M., Dunn, G., Meaden, A., Tarrier, N., Lewis, S., Wykes, T., Davies, L., Michail, M., & Peters, E. (2017). The COMMAND trial of cognitive therapy to prevent harmful compliance with command hallucinations: Predictors of outcome and mediators of change. *Psychological Medicine*, 1–9.

Birchwood, M., Gilbert, P., Gilbert, J., Trower, P., Meaden, A., Hay, J., Murray, E., & Miles, J. N. V. (2004). Interpersonal and role-related schema influence the relationship with the dominant "voice" in schizophrenia: A comparison of three models. *Psychological Medicine, 34*, 1–10.

Birchwood, M., Michail, M., Meaden, M., Tarrier, N., Lewis, S., Wykes, T., Davies, L., Dunn, G., & Peters, E. (2014). Cognitive behaviour therapy to prevent harmful compliance with command hallucinations (COMMAND): A randomised controlled trial. *Lancet Psychiatry, 1*, 23–33.

Birchwood, M., Spencer, E., & McGovern, D. (2000). Schizophrenia: Early warning signs. *Advances in Psychiatric Treatment, 6*(2), 93–101.

Blumenthal, S., & Lavender, T. (2000). *Violence and mental disorder: A critical aid to the assessment and management of risk*. Jessica Kingsley Publishers.

Blunden, R., & Allen, D. (1987). *Facing the challenge: An ordinary life for people with a learning disability and challenging behaviour* (Kings Fund Paper no. 74). Kings Fund Centre. www.nes.scot.nhs.uk/media/570730/pbs_interactive_final_nov_12.pdf

Bonta, J., Law, M., & Hanson, K. (1998). The prediction of criminal recidivism among disordered offenders: A meta-analysis. *Psychological Bulletin*, *123*(2), 123–142.

Bora, E., Yucel, M., & Pantelis, C. (2010). Cognitive impairment in schizophrenia and affective psychoses: Implications for DSM-V criteria and beyond. *Schizophrenia Bulletin*, *36*, 36–42.

Braithwaite, E., Charette, Y., Crocker, A. G., & Reyes, A. (2010). The predictive validity of clinical ratings of the short-term assessment of risk and treatability (START). *International Journal of Forensic Mental Health*, *9*(4), 271–281.

British Psychological Society. (2018). *Positive behavioural support*. Division of Clinical Psychology; Faculty for People with Intellectual Learning Disabilities. Retrieved March 23, 2020, from www.bps.org.uk/sites/www.bps.org.uk/files/Member%20Net works/Divisions/DCP/Positive%20Behaviour%20Support.pdf

Brown, S. (1997). Excess mortality of schizophrenia. *British Journal of Psychiatry*, *171*, 502–508.

Buchanan, A. (2008). Risk of violence by psychiatric patients: Beyond the "actuarial versus clinical" assessment debate. *Psychiatric Services*, *58*(2), 184–190.

Burns, T., Knapp, M., Catty, J., Healey, A., Henderson, J., Watt, H., & Wright, C. (2001). Home treatment for mental health problems: A systematic review. *Health Technological Assessment*, *5*(15).

Butler, G. (2006). The value of formulation: A question for debate. *Clinical Psychology Forum*, *41*, 36–40.

Carden, L. J., Saini, P., Seddon, C., Watkins, M., & James, T. P. (2018). Shame and the psychosis continuum: A systematic review of the literature. *Psychology & Psychotherapy: Theory, Research & Practice*. Advance online publication. https://doi.org/10.1111/papt.12204

Carpenter, R., Falkenburg, J., White, T., & Tracy, D. (2013). Crisis teams: Systematic review of their effectiveness in practice. *The Psychiatrist*, *37*(7), 232–237.

Carr, E. G., Carlson, J. I., Langdon, N. A., Magito-McLaughlin, D., & Yarbrough, C. C. (1998). Two perspectives on antecedent control: Molecular and molar. *Antecedent Control: Innovative Approach to Behavioural Support*, 3–28.

Cattell, V. (2001). Poor people, poor places, and poor health: The mediating role of social networks and social capital. *Social Science & Medicine*, *52*(10), 1501–1516.

Centre for Social Justice. (2011). *Completing the revolution: Transforming mental health and tackling poverty*. CSJ (In Johnson, S. (2013). Crisis resolution and home treatment teams: An evolving model. *Advances in Psychiatric Treatment*, *19*(2), 115–123).

Chadwick, P. (2006). *Person-based cognitive therapy for distressing psychosis*. Wiley.

Chadwick, P. (2014). Mindfulness for psychosis. *The British Journal of Psychiatry*, *204*(5), 333–334.

Chadwick, P., & Birchwood, M. (1994). The omnipotence of voices: A cognitive approach to auditory hallucinations. *British Journal of Psychiatry*, *164*, 190–201.

Chadwick, P., Birchwood, M., & Trower, P. (1996). *Cognitive therapy for delusions, voices and paranoia*. Wiley.

Chadwick, P., Lees, S., & Birchwood, M. (2000). The revised Beliefs About Voices Questionnaire (BAVQ-R). *British Journal of Psychiatry*, *177*, 229–232.

The Challenging Behaviour Foundation. (2014). *Information sheet; positive behavioural support planning: Part 3*. Retrieved June 1, 2020, from www.challengingbehaviour.org.uk/ learning-disability-files/03-Positive-Behaviour-Support-Planning-Part-3-web-2014.pdf

Cipani, E. (2018). *Functional behavioural assessment, diagnosis, and treatment* (3rd ed.). Springer.

Clifford, P., Leiper, R., Lavender, A., & Pilling, S. (1989). *Assuring quality in mental health services: The quartz system*. Free Association Books.

Copello, A., Williamson, E., Orford, J., & Day, E. (2006). Implementing and evaluating social behaviour and network therapy in drug treatment practice in the UK: A feasibility study. *Addictive Behaviors, 31*(5), 802–810.

Couture, S. M., Penn, D. L., & Roberts, D. L. (2006). The functional significance of social cognition in schizophrenia: A review. *Schizophrenia Bulletin, 32*(suppl_1), 44–63.

Cowan, C., Meaden, A., Commander, M., & Edwards, T. (2012). In-patient psychiatric rehabilitation services: Survey of service users in three metropolitan boroughs. *The Psychiatrist, 36*, 85–89.

Crisis Resolution Home Treatment (CRHT) Operational Policy. (2007).

Christofides, S., Johnstone, L., & Musa, M. (2012). "Chipping in": Clinical psychologists' descriptions of their use of formulation in multidisciplinary team working. *Psychology and Psychotherapy, 85*(4), 424–435.

Daffern, M., Howells, K., & Ogloff, J. R. P. (2007). The interaction between individual characteristics and the function of aggression in forensic psychiatric inpatients. *Psychiatry, Psychology and Law, 14*, 17–25.

Davies, B. D., Lowe, L., Morgan, S., John-Evans, H., & Fitoussi, J. (2019). An evaluation of the effectiveness of positive behavioural support within a medium secure mental health forensic service. *The Journal of Forensic Psychiatry and Psychology, 30*(1), 38–52.

Department of Health. (2007). *Best practice in managing risk*. Department of Health. https://assets.publishing.service.gov.uk/government/uploads/system/uploads/attachment_data/file/478595/best-practice-managing-risk-cover-webtagged.pdf

Department of Health. (2014). *Positive and proactive care: Reducing the need for restrictive interventions*. Retrieved April 4, 2020, from https://assets.publishing.service.gov.uk/government/uploads/system/uploads/attachment_data/file/300293/JRA_DoH_Guidance_on_RP_web_accessible.pdf

de Winter, C. F., Jansen, A. A. C., & Evenhuis, H. M. (2011). Physical conditions and challenging behaviour in people with intellectual disability: A systematic review. *Journal of Intellectual Disability Research, 55*(7), 675–698.

Division of Clinical Psychology. (2011). *Good practice guidelines on the use of psychological formulation*. British Psychological Society.

Docherty, J. P., Van Kammen, D. P., & Siris, S. G. (1978). Stages of onset of schizophrenic psychosis. *American Journal of Psychiatry, 135*, 420–426.

Douglas, K. S., Hart, S. D., Webster, C. D., & Belfrage, H. (2013). *HCR-20V3: Assessing risk of violence – user guide*. Mental Health, Law, and Policy Institute, Simon Fraser University.

Douglas, K. S., & Skeem, J. L. (2005). Violence risk assessment: Getting specific about being dynamic. *Psychology, Public Policy and Law, 11*(3), 347–383.

Edwards, T., Macpherson, R., Commander, M., Meaden, A., & Kalidindi, S. (2016). Services for people with complex psychosis: Towards a new understanding. *BJPsych Bulletin, 40*, 156–161.

Edwards, T., Meaden, A., & Commander, M. (2022). A ten year follow up service evaluation of the treatment pathway outcomes for patients in nine in-patient psychiatric rehabilitation services. *BJPsych Bulletin, 0,* 1–5.

Edwards, T., Macpherson, R., Commander, M., Meaden, A., & Kalidindi, S. (2016). Services for people with complex psychosis: Towards a new understanding *BJPsych Bulletin, 40,* 156–161.

Eells, T. D. (2007). Introduction. In T. D. Eells (Ed.), *Handbook of psychotherapy case formulation* (2nd ed., pp. 3–32). Guilford Press.

Eisler, R. M., Blanchard, E. B., Fitts, H., & Williams, J. G. (1978). Social skill training with and without modeling for schizophrenic and non-psychotic hospitalized psychiatric patients. *Behavior Modification, 2*(2), 147–172.

Elis, O., Caponigro, J. M., & Kring, A. M. (2013). Psychosocial treatments for negative symptoms in schizophrenia: Current practices and future directions. *Clinical Psychology Review, 33,* 914–928.

Ellis, A. (2004). *Reason and emotion in psychotherapy.* Lyle Stuart,.

Emerson, E. (2001). *Challenging behaviour: Analysis and intervention in people with learning difficulties* (2nd ed.). Cambridge University Press.

Emsley, R., Chiliza, B., Asmal, L., & Harvey, B. H. (2013). The nature of relapse in schizophrenia. *BMC Psychiatry, 13,* 50. https://doi.org/10.1186/1471-244X-13-50.

Emsley, R., Oosthuizen, P. P., Koen, L., Niehaus, D. J., & Martinez, G. (2012). Symptom recurrence following intermittent treatment in first-episode schizophrenia successfully treated for 2 years: A 3-year open-label clinical study. *Journal of Clinical Psychiatry, 73*(4), 541–547.

Eriksson, Å., Romelsjö, A., Stenbacka, M., & Tengström, A. (2011). Early risk factors for criminal offending in schizophrenia: A 35-year longitudinal cohort study. *Social Psychiatry and Psychiatric Epidemiology, 46,* 925–932.

Evans, N., & Whitcombe, S. (2015). Using circular questions as a tool in qualitative research. *Nurse Researcher, 23*(3), 28–31.

Fazel, S., Gulati, G., Linsell, L., Geddes, J. R., & Grann, M. (2009). Schizophrenia and violence: Systematic review and meta-analysis. *PLOS Medicine, 6*(8), e1000120. https://doi.org/10.1371/journal.pmed.1000120

Fett, A. J., Viechtbauer, W., Dominguez, M., Penn, D. L., van Os, J., & Krabbendam, L. (2011). The relationship between neurocognition and social cognition with functional outcomes in schizophrenia: A meta-analysis. *Neuroscience & Biobehavioral Reviews, 35,* 573–588.

Foussias, G., & Remington, G. (2010). Negative symptoms in schizophrenia: Avolition and Occam's razor. *Schizophrenia Bulletin, 36*(2), 359–369.

Fox, A., & Harrop, C. (2015). Enhancing social participation and recovery through a cognitive developmental approach. In A. Meaden & A. Fox (Eds.), *Innovations in psychosocial interventions for psychosis: Working with the hard to reach* (pp. 129–147). Routledge.

Fox, A., & Meaden, A. (2015). Team-based cognitive therapy for problematic behaviour associated with negative symptoms. In A. Meaden & A. Fox (Eds.), *Innovations in psychosocial interventions for psychosis: Working with the hard to reach* (pp. 219–233). Routledge.

Fox, A., & Sharp, R. (2018). *Dealing with stress: Psychology group manual.* NHS Mental Health Foundation Trust, Unpublished report.

Freeman, D., Taylor, K. M., Molodynski, A., & Waite, F. (2019). Treatable clinical intervention targets for patients with schizophrenia. *Schizophrenia Research, 211*, 44–50.

Gaebel, W., & Riesbeck, M. (2007). Revisiting the relapse predictive validity of prodromal symptoms in schizophrenia. *Schizophrenia Research, 95*(1–3), 19–29.

Gard, D. E., Kring, A. M., Gard, M. G., Horan, W. P., & Green, M. F. (2007). Anhedonia in schizophrenia: Distinctions between anticipatory and consummatory pleasure. *Schizophrneia Research, 93*, 253–260.

Geach, N., Mogaddham, N. G., & De Boos, D. (2018). A systematic review of team formulation in clinical psychology practice: Definition, implementation, and outcomes. *Psychology and Psychotherapy: Theory, Research and Practice, 91*, 186–215.

Gibson, S., Brand, S. L., Burt, S., Boden, Z. B. R., & Benson, O. (2013). Understanding treatment non-adherence in schizophrenia and bipolar disorder: A survey of what service users do and why. *BMC Psychiatry, 13*(1), 1–12.

Gilburt, H. (2018). *Funding and staffing of NHS mental health providers: Still waiting for parity.* www.kingsfund.org.uk/publications/funding-staffing-mental-health-providers

Gillespie, M. (2015). Adapting relapse-prevention strategies for use with difficult to engage populations. In A. Meaden & A. Fox (Eds.), *Innovations in psychosocial interventions for psychosis; working with the hard to reach.* Routledge.

Gore, N. J., McGill, P., Toogood, S., Allen, D., Hughes, C., Baker, P., Hastings, R. P., Noone, S., & Denne, L. (2013). Definition and scope for positive behaviour support. *International Journal of Positive Behavioural Support, 3*(2), 14–23.

Graham, H. L., Copello, A., Birchwood, M. J., Mueser, K., Orford, J., McGovern, D., Atkinson, E., Maslin, J., Preece, M., Tobin, D., & Georgiou, G. (2004). *Cognitive-behavioural integrated treatment (C-BIT): A treatment manual for substance misuse in people with severe mental health problems.* John Wiley & Sons Ltd.

Green, L. W. (2008). Making research relevant: If it is an evidence-based practice, where's the practice-based evidence?. *Family Practice, 25*(suppl 1), i20–i24.

Greenhalgh, T., Robert, G., Macfarlane, F., Bate, P., & Kyriakidou, O. (2004). Diffusion of innovations in service organizations: Systematic review and recommendations. *The Milbank Quarterly, 82*(4), 581–629.

Griffiths, R., & Harrias, N. (2008). The compatibility of psychosocial interventions (PSI) and assertive outreach: A survey of managers and PSI-trained staff in the UK assertive outreach teams. *Journal of Psychiatric and Mental Health Nursing, 15*, 479–483.

Habtewold, T. D., Rodijk, L. H., Liemburg, E. J., Sidorenkov, G., Boezen, H. M., Bruggeman, R., & Alizadeh, B. Z. (2020). A systematic review and narrative synthesis of data-driven studies in schizophrenia symptoms and cognitive deficits. *Translational Psychiatry, 10*(1), 1–24.

Hacker, D. A., Birchwood, M., Tudway, J., Meaden, A. T., & Amphlett, C. (2008). Acting on voices: Omnipotence, sources of threat and safety-seeking behaviours. *British Journal of Clinical Psychology, 47*(2), 201–203.

Haddock, G., Barrowclough, C., Shaw, J. J., Dunn, G., Novaco, R. W., & Tarrier, N. (2009). Cognitive–behavioural therapy v. social activity therapy for people with psychosis and a history of violence: Randomised controlled trial. *British Journal of Psychiatry, 194*, 152–157.

Haddock, G., Lowens, I., Brosnan, N., Barrowclough, C., & Novaco, R. W. (2004). Cognitive-behaviour therapy for inpatients with psychosis and anger problems within a low secure environment. *Behavioural and Cognitive Psychotherapy, 32*(1), 77–98.

Hanley, G. P. (2012). Functional assessment of problem behavior: Dispelling myths, overcoming implementation obstacles, and developing new lore. *Behavior Analysis in Practice*, *5*(1), 54–72.

Hanley, G. P., Iwata, B. A., & McCord, B. E. (2003). Functional analysis of problem behavior: A review. *Journal of Applied Behavior Analysis*, *36*(2), 147–185.

Hansen, L., Jones, R. M., & Kingdon, D. (2004). No Association between akathisia or parkinsonism and suicidality in treatment-resistant schizophrenia. *Journal of Psychopharmacology*, *18*(3), 384–387.

Hare-Duke, L., Dening, T., de Oliveira, D., Milner, K., & Slade, M. (2019). Conceptual framework for social connectedness in mental disorders: Systematic review and narrative synthesis. *Journal of Affective Disorders*, *245*, 188–199.

Hayes, L., & Coyne, L. (2021). *ACT conversations: Values cards for use in individual and group therapy with young people*. Retrieved October 24, 2021, from https://contextualscience.org/ louise_hayes_training_page

Hayward, M., Edgecumbe, R., Jones, A. M., Berry, C., & Strauss, C. (2018). Brief coping strategy enhancement for distressing voices: An evaluation in routine clinical practice. *Behavioural and Cognitive Psychotherapy*, *46*(2), 226–237.

Healthcare Commission. (2008). *The pathway to recovery: A review of acute inpatient mental health services*. Healthcare Commission (In Johnson, S. (2013). Crisis resolution and home treatment teams: An evolving model. *Advances in Psychiatric Treatment*, *19*(2), 115–123).

Hockenhull, J. C., Whittington, R., Leitner, M., Barr, W., & McGuire, J. (2012). A systematic review of prevention and intervention strategies for populations at high risk of engaging in violent behaviour. *Health Technology Assessment*, *16*(3), 1–152.

Hogg, L., & Hall, J. (1992). Management of long term impairments and challenging behaviour. In M. Birchwood & N. Tarrier (Eds.), *Innovations in the psychological management of schizophrenia: Assessment, treatment and services* (pp. 171–203). Wiley.

Holmes, J. (2004). What can psychotherapy contribute to improving the culture on acute wards. In P. Campling, S. Davies, & G. Farquharson (Eds.), *From toxic institutions to therapeutic environments: Residential settings in mental health services* (pp. 208–215). Gaskell.

Horan, W. P., & Green, M. F. (2019). Treatment of social cognition in schizophrenia: Current status and future directions. *Schizophrenia Research*, *203*, 3–11.

Horner, R. H., Dunlap, G., Koegel, R. L., Carr, E. G., Sailor, W., Anderson, J., Albin, R. W., & O'Neill, R. E. (1990). Toward a technology of "non-aversive" behavioural support. *Journal of the Association for Persons with Severe Handicaps*, *15*(3), 125–132.

Jansen, J. E., Gleeson, J., Bendall, S., Rice, S., & Alvarez-Jimenez, M. (2020). Acceptance- and mindfulness-based interventions for persons with psychosis: A systematic review and meta-analysis. *Schizophrenia Research*, *215*, 25–37.

Javed, A., & Charles, A. (2018). The importance of social cognition in improving functional outcomes in schizophrenia. *Frontiers in Psychiatry*, *9*, 157.

Johnstone, L. (2018). Psychological formulation as an alternative to psychiatric diagnosis. *Journal of Humanistic Psychology*, *58*(1), 30–46.

Joint Commissioning Panel for Mental Health. (2016). *Guidance for commissioners of rehabilitation services for people with complex mental health needs*. Joint Commissioning Panel for Mental Health. https://www.rcpsych.ac.uk/docs/default-source/members/faculties/rehabilitation-and-social-psychiatry/rehab-social—joint-commissioning-panel—guidance-for-commissioners-of-rehabilitation-servicesfor-people-with-complex-mental-health-needs—2016.pdf?sfvrsn=82cbb5e4_6

Jones, C., Hacker, D., Xia, J., Meaden, A., Irving, C. B., Zhao, S., Chen, J., & Shi, C. (2018). Cognitive behavioural therapy plus standard care versus standard care for people with schizophrenia. *Cochrane Database of Systematic Reviews, 12*, Art. No.: CD007964. https://doi.org/10.1002/14651858.CD007964.pub2

Kahneman, D., & Tversky, A. (1979). Prospect theory: An analysis of detection under risk. *Econometrica, 47*, 263–291.

Keet, R., de Vetten-Mc Mahon, M., Shields-Zeeman, L., Ruud, T., van Weeghel, J., Bahler, M., Mulder, C. L., Van Zelst, C., Murphy, B., Westen, K., & Nas, C. (2019). Recovery for all in the community; position paper on principles and key elements of community-based mental health care. *BMC Psychiatry, 19*, 174.

Keller, F. S., & Schoenfeld, W. N. (1950, 1995). *Principles of psychology: A systematic text in the science of behavior*. BF Skinner Foundation.

Killaspy, H., Bebbington, P., Blizard, R. Johnson, S., Nolan, F., Pilling, S., & King, M. (2006). The REACT study: Randomised evaluation of assertive community treatment in North. *British Medical Journal, 332*, 815. https://doi.org/10.1136/bmj.38773.518322.7C

Killaspy, H., Harden, C., Holloway, F., & King, M. (2005). What do mental health rehabilitation units do and what are they for? A national survey in England. *Journal of Mental Health, 14*, 157–165.

Killaspy, H., Marston, L., Green, N., Harrison, I., Lean, M., Cook, S., Mundy, T., Craig, T., Holloway, F., Leavey, G., & Koeser, L. (2015). Clinical effectiveness of a staff training intervention in mental health inpatient rehabilitation units designed to increase patients' engagement in activities (the rehabilitation effectiveness for activities for life [REAL] study): Single-blind, cluster-randomised controlled trial. *Lancet Psychiatry, 2*, 38–48.

Kiresuk, T. J., Smith, A., & Cardillo, J. E. (1994). *Goal attainment scale: Applications, theory and measurement*. Lawrence Erlbaum Associates, Inc.

Kirschner, M., Aleman, A., & Kaiser, S. (2017). Secondary negative symptoms: A review of mechanisms, assessment and treatment. *Schizophrenia Research, 186*, 29–38.

Knight, M. T. D., Wykes, T., & Hayward, P. (2003). "People don't understand": An investigation of stigma in schizophrenia using interpretative phenomenological analysis (IPA). *Journal of Mental Health, 12*, 209–222.

Kurtz, M. M., & Richardson, C. L. (2012). Social cognitive training for schizophrenia: A meta-analytic investigation of controlled research. *Schizophrenia Bulletin, 38*, 1092–1104.

Kuyken, W. (2006). Evidence-based case formulation: Is the emperor clothed? In N. Tarrier (Ed.), *Case formulation in cognitive behaviour therapy: The treatment of challenging and complex cases* (pp. 12–35). Routledge.

Lake, N. (2008). Developing skills in consultation 2: A team formulation approach. *Clinical Psychology Forum, 186*, 18–24.

Lamothe, J., Boyer, R., & Guay, S. (2021). A longitudinal analysis of psychological distress among healthcare workers following patient violence. *Canadian Journal of Behavioural Science/Revue canadienne des sciences du comportement, 53*(1), 48–58.

Lavender, A. (1984). *Evaluation in settings for the long term psychologically handicapped. Unpublished* [PhD thesis, Kings College Hospital Medical School, University of London].

Lavender, A. (1987). The measurement of the quality of care in psychiatric rehabilitation settings: Development of the model standards questionnaires. *Behavioral Psychotherapy, 15*, 201–214.

Lavender, A., Leiper, R., Pilling, S., & Clifford, P. (1994). Quality assurance in mental health: The QUARTZ system. *British Journal of Clinical Psychology*, *33*, 451–476.

LaVigna, G. W., & Donnellan, A. M. (1986). *Alternatives to punishment: Solving behaviour problems with non-aversive strategies*. Irvington Inc.

LaVigna, G. W., Willis, T. J., & Donnellan, A. M. (1989). The role of positive programming in behavioral treatment. In E. Cippani (Ed.), *The treatment of severe behavior disorders: Behavior analysis approaches*. AAMR.

Large, M. M., & Ryan, C. J. (2014). "Heed not the oracle": Risk assessment has no role in preventing suicide in schizophrenia. *Acta Psychiatrica Scandinavica*, *130*, 415–417.

Lee, S. H., Choi, T. K., Suh, S., Kim, Y. W., Kim, B., Lee, E., & Yook, K. H. (2010). The effectiveness of a psychosocial intervention for relapse prevention in patients with schizophrenia receiving risperidone via long-acting injection. *Psychiatry Research*, *175*, 195–199.

Leff, J., & Szmidla, A. (2002). Evaluation of a special rehabilitation programme for patients who are difficult to place. *Social Psychiatry and Psychiatric Epidemiology*, *37*, 532–536.

Lelliott, P., Audini, B., Knapp, M., & Chisholm, D. (1996). The mental health residential care study: Classification of facilities and description of residents. *The British Journal of Psychiatry*, *169*, 139–147.

Lidz, C., Mulvey, E., & Gardner, W. (1993). The accuracy of predictions of violence to others. *Journal of the American Medical Association*, *269*, 1007–1011.

Linszen, D., Lenior, M., & de Haan, L. (1998). Early intervention, untreated psychosis and the course of early schizophrenia. *British Journal of Psychiatry*, *172*(suppl 33), 84–89.

Lobban, F., Taylor, L., Chandler, E., Tyler, E., Kinderman, P., Kolamunnage-Donna, R., Gamble, C., Peters, S., Pontin, E., Sellwood, W., & Morriss, R. K. (2010). Enhanced relapse prevention for bipolar disorder by community mental health teams: Cluster feasibility randomised trial. *British Journal of Psychiatry*, *196*, 59–63.

Lucre, K., & Clapton, N. (2021). The compassionate kitbag: A creative and integrative approach to compassion-focused therapy. *Psychology and Psychotherapy: Theory, Research and Practice*, *94*, 497–516.

Lutgens, D., Gariepy, G., & Malla, A. (2017). Psychological and psychosocial interventions for negative symptoms in psychosis: Systematic review and meta-analysis. *The British Journal of Psychiatry*, *210*(5), 324–332.

Lynch, M. A. (2014). *Exploring the understanding and use of "case busts" within two assertive outreach teams*. https://etheses.bham. ac.uk //id/eprint/5372/1/ Lynch14 MRes. pdf.

Lyons, C., Hopley, P., & Burton, C. R. (2009). Mental health crisis and respite services: Service user and carer aspirations. *Journal of Psychiatric and Mental Health Nursing*, *16*, 424–433.

Marriott, R., O'Shea, L. E., Picchioni, M. M., & Dickens, G. L. (2017). Predictive validity of the short-term assessment of risk and treatability (START) for multiple adverse outcomes: The effect of diagnosis. *Psychiatry Research*, *25*(6), 435–443.

McDonald, S. (2012). New frontiers in neuropsychological assessment: Assessing social perception using a standardised instrument, the awareness of social inference test. *Australian Psychologist*, *47*(1), 39–48.

McDonnell, A. A. (1999). Defusing violent situations: Low arousal approaches. *British Journal of Therapy and Rehabilitation*, *6*(2), 71–74.

McDonnell, A. A., Reeves, S., Johnson, A., & Lane, A. (1998). Managing challenging behaviour in an adult with learning disabilities: The use of low arousal approach. *Behavioural and Cognitive Psychotherapy, 26*(2), 163–171.

McTiernan, K., Jackman, L., Robinson, L., & Thomas, M. (2021). A thematic analysis of the multidisciplinary team understanding of the 5P team formulation model and its evaluation on a psychosis rehabilitation unit. *Community Mental Health Journal, 57*, 579–588.

Meaden, A., Commander, M., Edwards, T., & Cowan, C. (2014). Patient engagement and problematic behaviours in residential rehabilitation units. *Psychiatric Bulletin, 38*, 260–264.

Meaden, A., Fox, A., & Hacker, D. A. (2015). Team-based cognitive therapy for distress and problematic behaviour associated with positive symptoms. In A. Meaden & A. Fox (Eds.), *Innovations in psychosocial interventions for psychosis: Working with the hard to reach* (pp. 184–199). Routledge.

Meaden, A., & Hacker, D. A. (2010). *Risk and problematic behaviour in psychosis: A shared formulation approach.* Routledge.

Meaden, A., Hacker, D. A., & Spencer, K. (2013). Acute aggression risk: An early warning signs methodology. *Journal of Forensic Practice, 15*(1), 21–31.

Meaden, A., Hacker, D. A., Villiers, A., Carbourne, J., & Paget, A. (2012). Developing a measurement of engagement: The residential rehabilitation engagement scale for psychosis. *Journal of Mental Health, 21*(2), 182–191.

Meaden, A., & Hewson, H. (2015). Long-term supportive psychotherapy as a team based therapy. In A. Meaden & A. Fox (Eds.), *Innovations in psychosocial interventions for psychosis: Working with the hard to reach.* Routledge.

Meaden, A., & Kalidindi, S. (2015). A comprehensive approach to assessment in rehabilitation settings. In G. Roberts, S. Davenport, F. Holloway, & T. Tattan (Eds.), *Enabling recovery: The principles and practice of rehabilitation psychiatry* (2nd ed.). Gaskell.

Meaden, A., Keen, N., Aston, R., Barton, K., & Bucci, S. (2013). *Cognitive therapy for command hallucinations: An advanced practical companion.* Routledge.

Meehl, P. (1954). *Clinical versus statistical prediction: A theoretical analysis and a review of the evidence.* University of Minnesota Press.

Millon, T. (1997). *MCMI-III: Manual.* NCS Pearson, Inc.

Mind. (2011). *Listening to experience: An independent report into acute and crisis mental healthcare.* Mind (In Johnson, S. (2013). Crisis resolution and home treatment teams: An evolving model. *Advances in Psychiatric Treatment, 19*(2), 115–123).

Monahan, J., Steadman, H. J., Silver, E., Appelbaum, P. S., Robbins, P. C., Mulvey, E., Roth, L., Grisso, T., & Banks, S. (2001). *Rethinking risk assessment: The MacArthur study of mental disorder and violence.* Oxford University Press.

Morgan, S. (1998). The assessment and management of risk. In C. Brooker & J. Repper (Eds.), *Serious mental health problems in the community: Policy, practice and research* (pp. 265–290). Bailliere Tindall.

Moritz, S., Veckenstedt, R., Bohn, F., Köther, U., & Woodward, T. S. (2013). Metacognitive training in schizophrenia: Theoretical rationale and administration. In D. L. Roberts & D. L. Penn (Eds.), *Social cognition in schizophrenia.* Oxford University Press.

Moritz, S., & Woodward, T. S. (2005). Jumping to conclusions in delusional and non-delusional schizophrenic patients. *British Journal of Clinical Psychology, 44*(2), 193–207.

Murphy, S., Osborne, H., & Smith, I. (2013). Psychological consultation in older adult inpatient settings: A qualitative investigation of the impact on staff's daily practice and the mechanisms of change. *Aging and Mental Health, 17*(4), 441–448.

National Audit Office. (2007). *Helping people through mental health crisis: The role of crisis resolution and home treatment teams.* National Audit Office (In Johnson, S. (2013). Crisis resolution and home treatment teams: An evolving model. *Advances in Psychiatric Treatment, 19*(2), 115–123).

National Institute for Health and Care Excellence (NICE). (2014). *Psychosis and schizophrenia in adults: Prevention and management.* Retrieved September 21, 2021, from www.nice.org.uk/ guidance/ cg178/chapter/1-Recommendations#subsequent-acute-episodes-of-psychosis-or-schizophrenia-and-referral-in-crisis-2

NHS (The NHS Long Term Plan). 2019. *Royal college of psychiatry getting it right first time.* www.gettingitrightfirsttime.co.uk/virtual-visits-begin-as-girft-mental-health-rehabilitation-review-gets-under-way

O'Shea, L. E., & Dickens, G. L. (2014). Short-term assessment of risk and treatability (START): Systematic review and meta-analysis. *Psychological Assessment, 26*(3), 990–1002.

O'Shea, L. E., Picchioni, M. M., & Dickens, G. L. (2016). The predictive validity of the short-term assessment of risk and treatability (START) for multiple adverse outcomes in a secure psychiatric inpatient setting. *Assessment, 23*(2), 150–162.

Palmer, B. W., Dawes, S. E., & Heaton, R. K. (2009). What do we know about neuropsychological aspects of schizophrenia? *Neuropsychological Review, 19*, 365–384.

Papadopoulos, A., Fox, A., & Herriott, M. (2013). Recovering wellbeing: An integrative framework. *British Journal of Mental Health Nursing, 2*(3), 145–154.

Peters, S., Pontin, E., Lobban, F., & Morriss, R. (2011). Involving relatives in relapse prevention for bipolar disorder: A multi-perspective qualitative study of value and barriers. *BMC Psychiatry, 172.* https://doi.org/10.1186/1471-244X-11-172

Peterson, J. K., Skeem, J., Kennealy, P., Bray, B., & Zvonkovic, A. (2014). How often and how consistently do symptoms directly precede criminal behavior among offenders with mental illness? *Law and Human Behavior, 38*(5), 439–449

Pfammatter, M., Brenner, H. D., Junghan, U. M., & Tschacher, W. (2011). The importance of cognitive processes for the integrative treatment of persons with schizophrenia. *Schizophrenia Bulletin, 37*(suppl 2), S1–S4.

Pompili, M., Amador, X. F., Girardi, P., Harkavy-Friedman, J., Harrow, M., Kaplan, K., Krausz, M., Lester, D., Meltzer, H. Y., Modestin, J., & Montross, L. P. (2007). Suicide risk in schizophrenia: Learning from the past to change the future. *Annals of General Psychiatry, 6*, 10. https://doi.org/10.1186/1744-859X-6-10

Pontin, E., Peters, S., Lobban, F., Rogers, A., & Morriss, R. K. (2009). Enhanced relapse prevention for bipolar disorder: A qualitative investigation of value perceived for service users and care coordinators. *Implementation Science.* https://doi.org/10.1186/1748-5908-4-4

Popovic, D., Benabarre, A., Crespo, J. M., Goikolea, J. M., González-Pinto, A., Gutiérrez-Rojas, L., Montes, J. M., & Vieta, E. (2014). Risk factors for suicide in schizophrenia: Systematic review and clinical recommendations. *Acta Psychiatrica Scandinavica, 130*(6), 418–426.

Powell, J., Geddes, J., & Hawton, K. (2000). Suicide in psychiatric hospital in-patients: Risk factors and their predictive power. *The British Journal of Psychiatry, 176*, 266–272.

Quinsey, V. L., Harris, G. T., Rice, M. E., & Cormier, C. (1998). *Violent offenders: Appraising and managing risk.* American Psychological Association.

Quinsey, V. L., Jones, G. B., Book, A. S., & Barr, A. N. (2006). The dynamic prediction of antisocial behaviour among forensic psychiatric patients: A prospective field study. *Journal of Interpersonal Violence, 21*, 539–565.

Rector, N. A., Beck, A. T., & Stolar, N. (2005). The negative symptoms of schizophrenia: A cognitive perspective. *Canadian Journal of Psychiatry*, *50*, 247–257.

Reid, K. (2019). Is adjunctive CBT really effective for schizophrenia?: Commentary on . . . Cochrane corner. *BJPsych Advances*, *25*(5), 273–278.

Reser, M. P., Slikboer, R., & Rossell, S. I. (2019). A systematic review of factors that influence the efficacy of cognitive remediation therapy in schizophrenia. *Australian and & New Zealand Journal of Psychiatry*, *53*(7), 624–641.

Roberts, D. L., Penn, D. L., & Combs, D. R. (2016). *Social cognition and interaction training*. Oxford University Press.

Robinson, D. G., Woerner, M. G., Alvir, J. M., Bilder, R., Goldman, R., & Geisler, S. (1999). Predictors of relapse following response from a first episode of schizophrenia or schizoaffective disorder. *Archives of General Psychiatry*, *56*(3), 241–247.

Robinson, D. G., Woerner, M. G., McMeniman, M., Mendelowitz, A., & Bilder, R. M. (2004). Symptomatic and functional recovery from a first episode of schizophrenia or schizoaffective disorder. *American Journal of Psychiatry*, *161*, 473–479.

Robson, J., & Quayle, G. (2009). Increasing the utility of psychological formulation: A case example from an acute mental health ward. *Clinical Psychology Forum*, *204*, 25–29.

Rogers, P. (2004). *Command hallucinations and violence: Secondary analysis of the macarthur violence risk assessment data* [Unpublished doctoral dissertation, Institute of Psychiatry, Kings College].

Rogers, P. (2005). *The association between command hallucinations and prospective violence: Secondary analysis of the MacArthur violence risk assessment study* (Conference presentation). Institute of Psychiatry.

Royal College of Psychiatrists. (2007). *Accreditation for acute inpatient mental health services (AIMS): Pilot phase report*. www.rcpsych.ac.uk/pdf/AIMS%20Pilot%20Phase%20Report.pdf

Royal College of Psychiatrists. (2009). *Enabling recovery for people with mental health needs; a template for rehabilitation services* (Faculty report FR/RS/1). Royal College of Psychiatrists.

Royal College of Psychiatrists, British Psychological Society, Royal College of Speech and Language Therapists. (2007). *Challenging behaviour: A unified approach (CR144)*. www.rcpsych.ac.uk/ files/pdfversion/cr144.pdf

Saeri, A. K., Cruwys, T., Barlow, F. K., Stronge, S., & Sibley, C. G. (2018). Social connectedness improves public mental health: Investigating bidirectional relationships in the New Zealand attitudes and values survey. *Australian & New Zealand Journal of Psychiatry*, *52*(4), 365–374.

Sambrook, S. (2008). Working with crisis: The role of the clinical psychologist in a psychiatric intensive care unit. In I. Clarke & H. Wilson (Eds.), *Cognitive behaviour therapy for acute inpatient mental health units: Working with clients, staff and the milieu* (pp. 129–143). Routledge.

Schablon, A., Zeh, A., Wendeler, D., Peters, C., Wohlert, C., Harling, M., & Nienhaus, A. (2012). Frequency and consequences of violence and aggression towards employees in the German healthcare and welfare system: A cross-sectional study. *BMJ Open*, *2*(5), e001420, pmid:23087013

The Schizophrenia Commission. (2016). *Progress report: Five years on*. Rethink.

Shah, A., & Ganesvaran, T. (1999). Suicide among psychiatric in-patients with schizophrenia in an Australian mental hospital. *Medicine, Science and the Law*, *39*(3), 251–259.

Shepherd, A., Doyle, M., Sanders, C., & Shaw, J. (2016). Personal recovery within forensic settings – systematic review and meta-synthesis of qualitative methods studies. *Criminal Behaviour and Mental Health, 26*(1), 59–75.

Short, V., Covey, J. A., Webster, L. A., Wadman, R., Reilly, J., Hay-Gibson, N., & Stain, H. J. (2019). Considering the team in team formulation: A systematic review. *Mental Health Review Journal, 24*(1), 11–29.

Simó-Pinatella, D., Font-Roura, J., Alomar-Kurz, E., Giné, C., Matson, J. L., & Cifre, I. (2013). Antecedent events as predictive variables for behavioral function. *Research in Developmental Disabilities, 34*(12), 4582–4590.

Simpson, A. I., & Penney, S. R. (2018). Recovery and forensic care: Recent advances and future directions. *Criminal Behaviour and Mental Health, 28*, 383.

Simpson, A. J. O. (2019). *Identifying the needs of people with complex and enduring psychosis* [Unpublished master's thesis, University of Birmingham].

Singh, S. P. (2000). Running an effective community mental health team. *Advances in Psychiatric Treatment, 6*, 414–422.

Skeem, L., & Monahan, J. (2011). Current directions in violence risk assessment. *Current Directions in Psychological Science, 20*, 38–42.

Skills for Care & Skills for Health. (2014). *A positive and proactive workforce: A guide to workforce development for commissioners and employers seeking to minimise the use of restrictive practices in social care and health*. Retrieved April 4, 2020, from www.skillsforhealth.org.uk/images/projects/physical/A%20positive%20and%20proactive%20workforce.pdf

Skinner, B. F. (1971). *Beyond freedom and dignity*. Alfred A. Knopf.

Skinner, P., & Toogood, R. (Eds.). (2010). *Clinical psychology leadership development framework*. British Psychological Society.

Slade, M., Amering, M., Farkas, M., Hamilton, B., O'Hagan, M., Panther, G., & Whitley, R. (2014). Uses and abuses of recovery: Implementing recovery-oriented practices in mental health systems. *World Psychiatry, 13*(1), 12–20.

Swartz, M. S., Swanson, J. W., Hiday, V. A., Borum, R., & Wagner, R. (1998). Violence and severe mental illness: The effects of substance abuse and nonadherence to medication. *American Journal of Psychiatry, 155*, 226–231.

Swanson, J. W., Borum, R., Swartz, M. S., & Monahan, J. (1996). Psychotic symptoms and disorders and the risk of violent behavior in the community. *Criminal Behaviour and Mental Health, 6*, 309–329.

Swanson, J. W., Holzer, C. E., Ganju, V. K., & Jono, R. T. (1990). Violence and psychiatric disorder in the community: Evidence from the epidemiologic catchment area surveys. *Hospital and Community Psychiatry, 41*, 761–770.

Taylor, K. N., & Sambrook, S. (2012). CBT for culture change: Formulating teams to improve patient care. *Behavioural and Cognitive Psychotherapy, 40*(4), 496–503.

Teague, G. B., Bond, G. R., &Drake, R. E. (1998). Program fidelity in assertive community treatment: Development and use of a measure. *American Journal of Orthopsychiatry, 68*, 216–232.

Thorndike, E. L. (1911). Animal intelligence. In C. D. Green (Ed.), *Classics in the history of psychology*. http://psychclassics.yorku.ca/Thorndike/Animal/ chap5.htm

Tolisano, P., Sondik, T. M., & Dike, C. C. (2017). A positive behavioral approach for aggression in forensic psychiatric settings. *Journal of the American Academy of Psychiatry and the Law, 45*(1), 31–39.

Trower, P., Birchwood, M., Meaden, A., Byrne, S., Nelson, A., & Ross, K. (2004). Cognitive therapy for command hallucinations: Randomised controlled trial. *British Journal of Psychiatry*, *184*, 312–320.

Trower, P., & Chadwick, P. (1995). Pathways to defense of the self: A theory of two types of paranoia. *Clinical Psychology: Science and Practice*, *2*(3), 263.

Turton, P., Wright, C., White, S., & Killaspy, H. (2010). Promoting recovery in long-term institutional mental health care: An international Delphi Study. *Psychiatric Services*, *61*(3), 293–299. https://doi.org/10.1176/ps.2010.61.3.293

Van Os, J., Hanssen, M., Bijl, R. V., & Ravelli, A. (2000). Strauss (1969) revisited: A psychosis continuum in the general population? *Schizophrenia Research*, *45*, 11–20.

Varnik, P. (2012). Suicide in the world. *International Journal of Environmental Research and Public Health*, *9*, 760–771.

Velligan, D. I., Mahurin, R. K., Diamond, P. L., Hazleton, B. C., Eckert, S. L., & Miller, A. L. (1997). The functional significance of symptomatology and cognitive function in schizophrenia. *Schizophrenia Research*, *25*(1), 21–31.

Vigod, S. N., Kurdyak, P. A., Dennis, C. L., Leszcz, T., Taylor, V. H., & Blumberger, D. M. (2013). Transitional interventions to reduce early psychiatric readmissions in adults: Systematic review. *British Journal of Psychiatry*, *202*(3), 187–194.

Vigod, S. N., Kurdyak, P. A., Seitz, D., Herrman, N., Fung, K., & Lin, E. (2015). READMIT: A clinical risk index to predict 30-day readmission after discharge from acute psychiatric units. *Journal of Psychiatric Research*, *61*, 205–213.

Viljoen, J. L., Beneteau, J. L., Gulbransen, E., Brodersen, E., Desmarais, S. L., Nicholls, T. L., & Cruise, K. R. (2012). Assessment of multiple risk outcomes, strengths, and change with the START: A short-term prospective study with adolescent offenders. *International Journal of Forensic Mental Health*, *11*(3), 165–180.

Villanueva, J., Meyer, A. H., Rinner, M. T., Firsching, V. J., Benoy, C., Brogli, S., & Gloster, A. T. (2019). "Choose change": Design and methods of an acceptance and commitment therapy effectiveness trial for transdiagnostic treatment-resistant patients. *BMC Psychiatry*, *19*(1), 1–12.

Waite, F., Sheaves, B., Isham, L., Reeve, S., & Freeman, D. (2020). Sleep and schizophrenia: From epiphenomenon to treatable causal target. *Schizophrenia Research*, *221*, 44–56.

Wakefield, J. R. H., Kellezi, B., Stevenson, C., McNamara, N., Bowe, M., Wilson, I., & Mair, E. (2020). Social prescribing as "social cure": A longitudinal study of the health benefits of social connectedness within a social prescribing pathway. *Journal of Health Psychology*. https://doi.org/10.1177/1359105320944991

Ward, T., & Beech, A. R. (2004). The etiology of risk: A preliminary model. *Sexual Abuse: Journal of Research and Treatment*, *16*(4), 271–284.

Watt, D. C., Katz, K., & Shepard, M. (1983). The natural history of schizophrenia: A 5-year prospective follow-up of a Dutch incidence cohort. *Schizophrenia Bulletin*, *24*, 78–85.

Webster, C. D., Martin, M., Brink, J., Nicholls, T. L., & Middleton, C. (2004). *Short-term assessment of risk and treatability (START)*. St. Josephs Healthcare, Hamilton and British Columbia Mental Health and Addiction Services.

Webster, C. D., Nicholls, T. L., Martin, M. L., Desmarais, S. L., & Brink, J. (2006). Short-term assessment of risk and treatability (START): The case for a new structured professional judgment scheme. *Behavioral Sciences & the Law*, *24*(6), 747–766.

Westra, H. A., Aviram, A., & Doell, F. K. (2011). Extending motivational interviewing to the treatment of major mental health problems: Current directions and evidence. *The Canadian Journal of Psychiatry*, *56*(11), 643–650.

Whittington, R. (1994). Violence in psychiatric hospitals. In T. Wykes (Ed.), *Violence and mental health care professionals*. Chapman and Hall.

Wiersma, D., Nienhuis, F. J., Slooff, C. J., & Giel, R. (1998). Natural course of schizophrenic disorders: A 15-year follow up of a Dutch incidence cohort. *Schizophrenia Bulletin, 24*(1), 75–85.

Wilcox, E. (2013). Biscuits and perseverance: Reflections on supporting a community intellectual disability team to reflect. *Advances in Mental Health and Intellectual Disabilities, 7*(4), 211–219.

Williams, C. H. J. (2008). Cognitive behavioural therapy within assertive outreach teams: Barriers to implementation: A qualitative peer audit. *Journal of Psychiatric and Mental Health Nursing, 15*, 850–856.

Witt, K., van Dorn, R., & Fazel, S. (2013). Risk factors for violence in psychosis: Systematic review and meta-regression analysis of 110 studies. *PLOS ONE, 8*(2), e55942. https://doi.org/10.1371/journal.pone.0055942

Wolfesnsberger, W. (1983). Social role valorisation: A proposed new term for the principle of normalization. *Mental Retarded Journal, 9*(1), 4–11.

Wood, L., & Irons, C. (2016). Exploring the associations between social rank and external shame with experiences of psychosis. *Behavioural and Cognitive Psychotherapy, 44*(5), 527.

Wykes, T., Huddy, V., Cellard, C., McGurk, S. R., & Czobor, P. (2011). A meta-analysis of cognitive remediation for schizophrenia: Methodology and effect sizes. *American Journal of Psychiatry, 168*, 472–85.

Wykes, T., & Reeder, C. (2006). *Cognitive remediation therapy for schizophrenia: Theory and practice*. Routledge.

Young, J., Poole, U., Mohamed, F., Jian, S., Williamson, M., Ross, J., Jaye, C., Radue, P., & Egan, T. (2021). Exploring the value of social network 'care maps' in the provision of long-term conditions care. *Chronic Illness, 17*(2), 95–110.

Zubin, J., & Spring, B. (1977). Vulnerability: A new view of schizophrenia. *Journal of Abnormal Psychology, 86*(2), 103–126.

Index

5Ps 25

ABC: behavioural 75, 89, 96–97; cognitive
31–32, 35, 82, 105–106, 109–114, 120,
126, 128; of risk 13–15, 26
abuse 8, 13, 54, 66, 67, 70, 77–79, 162,
167–168, 170
Acceptance and Commitment Therapy
see ACT
ACT 129, 137
active behaviours 8, 62, 66, 72, 82–83, 93,
105, 129; *see also* problem behaviours;
active resistance behaviours 8, 13,
83; aims, stages and techniques for
107–112; CARM template for 196;
EWS-R for 62–64
activities of daily living *see* ADL
acute risk 13, 19, 43, 62, 71
ADHD 74, 145, 153
ADL 86, 115, 120, 153, 176–177
aggression 2, 11, 40, 73–74, 136; physical
1, 6–7, 38, 43, 52, 59, 64–65, 68, 79,
102, 121, 162–163, 177, 187, *see also*
violence; verbal 7, 38, 43, 59, 65–66,
70, 73–74, 85, 112, 121, 138, 154, 177,
184, 187
AIMS accreditation 24
alcohol 10, 14, 48, 61, 64, 79–81,
144–145, 147, 152–157, 164, 166
Allen, D. 5
amber behaviour 78, 96–98, 100–101, 178
anamnestic assessment 39
Andrews, D. A. 95
anger 33, 59, 67, 70, 91, 127, 133, 136,
151–152, 164, 166, 198
anhedonia 115–116
Antecedent-Behaviour-Consequence
see behavioural ABC

antisocial behaviour 6–7, 10, 31, 55, 66,
110, 124, 145, 147, 164–165
anxiety 10, 14, 60, 76, 88, 91, 103, 110,
122–124, 127, 130, 133–134, 163,
165–167, 171
AOTs 2–3, 23, 59, 122–123, 164
arson 6, 32, 38
Assertive Outreach Teams *see* AOTs
Attention Deficit Hyperactivity Disorder
74, 145, 153
attention seeking 8, 74, 93
attitudes (START area) 42, 49, 149, 164,
185
attribution biases 131–132
auditory hallucinations 9, 31, 52–54, 59,
62–63, 77–78, 84, 86, 107–108, 162,
164, 168–170
autism spectrum disorders 19
aversive care response 89–91
avoidance 60, 83, 86–87, 89–90, 94, 121,
124, 126, 131–133, 136
avolition 82, 115–116, 118
Awareness of Social Inference Test
131–132, 176
away days 18, 22, 24

Ballatt, J. 140
barriers to change 16–18
barriers to recovery 4, 24, 34, 55, 57, 72,
94, 104, 105, 108, 126, 142, 146, 161,
182
Beck, A. T. 82, 116, 118
Beech, A. R. 33, 41
behavioural ABC 75, 89, 96–97
behavioural deficits 7, 32, 36, 82, 177;
see also passive behaviours
behavioural experiments 120, 128, 130,
135

behavioural interventions 26, 55, 90, 92–104, 126, 128, 135, 152–153, 198
Beliefs About Voices Questionnaire 176
Bellack, A. S. 133
Bennett, R. 32
Bernard, M. 134
Berry, K. 25
bipolar disorder 185
Birchwood, M. 11, 13, 31, 125
blue behaviour 96, 99–101
Blunden, R. 5
British Psychological Society 29
burnout 21, 90, 139–140, 161

CAB framework 108, 120
Calgary Depression Scale 176
Campling, P. 140
care maps 140
care planning using multiple shared formulations 142–159
CARM 5–6, 17, 26, 31–36, 52–55, 65–66, 72–91, 95–96, 104, 105, 109, 111, 113, 116–119, 123–128, 135–136, 140–141, 143, 151, 153, 169–170, 174, 188; components of 76–79, *see also individual components*; developments in utilising 82–83; form and function 74–75; identifying factors for formulation 89, 91; importance of considering internal events 88; importance of operationalising the definition 73–74; order and process of collecting the information 88–89; principles of functional assessment 75–76; templates 196–197
Carpenter, R. 167
case coordination and recording 20
CBC-P 7, 13, 23, 26, 44, 177, 181, 188
CBRS-P 64, 68, 71, 97, 100–101, 103–104, 199
CBT 105, 117, 130, 134
CBT-P 1–2, 41, 58, 106, 115, 119–120, 125, 134, 190
Centre for Social Justice 167
CFT 165, 169
Chadwick, P. 11, 31
challenging behaviour 5–8, 93; *see also* problem behaviours
Challenging Behaviour Checklist for Psychosis *see* CBC-P
Challenging Behaviour Foundation 96
Challenging Behaviour Record Sheet for Psychosis *see* CBRS-P
child prostitution 77

Christofides, S. 22–23
Cipani, E. 76
Clifford, P. 18, 23
clinical judgement 32, 39, 62, 198; *see also* START
Clinician-Rated Outcome Measures 75, 177
clozapine 102
CMHTs 160–165, 167–168, 172, 174
cognitive ABC 31–32, 35, 82, 107, 109–111, 113–116, 122, 125, 129, 131
Cognitive Approach to Risk Management *see* CARM
Cognitive Behaviour Therapy *see* CBT
Cognitive Behaviour Therapy for Psychosis *see* CBT-P
cognitive biases 52, 106
cognitive deficits 31, 62, 117–118, 122, 124, 131, 138–139, 176
cognitive processing and behaviour 131–134
cognitive remediation therapy 131
Cognitive-Behavioural Integrated Treatment 159
command hallucinations 6, 9, 11, 40–42, 88, 105, 121, 165
Community Mental Health Teams *see* CMHTs
Community Rehabilitation Units *see* CRUs
compulsive behaviours 7, 13, 177
conduct (START area) 42, 50, 150, 164, 185
coping strategies 6, 39, 41, 43, 51, 58–60, 64, 68, 134, 151–152, 157, 159, 165–166, 198, 202
Couture, S. M. 131
COVID-19 pandemic 138, 161
Cowan, C. 1, 13
criminality 9–10, 39, 49, 66, 144–145, 147, 149, 152, 162, 165
cross-sectional formulation 31–32
CRUs 79, 137–138, 153–154

Dartmouth Assertive Community Treatment Scale 24
delusions 10, 13, 31–32, 40, 42, 47, 66, 70, 75–76, 78, 91, 102, 115–116, 118–119, 136, 144, 148, 198
Department of Health 39
depression 11, 157, 198
diabetes 31, 66, 69, 84, 115, 145, 186
discharge from service 2, 20, 40, 123–125, 133

distress 4, 10–11, 19, 23, 30–31, 40, 63, 79, 106–109, 113, 119, 125, 126–131, 136, 139–141, 189, 191
Docherty, J. P. 57
Donnellan, A. M. 93
Douglas, K. S. 5, 41
drug use *see* substance misuse

early warning signs 57–71, 78, 83, 98, 116, 118; *see also* EWS-P; EWS-R
Early Warning Signs of Psychotic Relapse *see* EWS-P
Early Warning Signs of Risk *see* EWS-R
Edwards, T. 2
Emerson, E. 5
emotional state (START area) 42, 47, 149, 156, 159, 164, 185
emotions, awareness and management of 133–134
empathy 35, 72, 74
engagement 2, 4, 23, 39, 59, 60–62, 136, 162–164, 176–177
Eriksson, Å. 9
escorted leave 65, 102, 145, 147
establishing operations 77–78, 82–83, 89–91, 127
Evans, N. 110
EWS-P 57–59, 62–64, 78, 113, 165
EWS-R 26, 33, 36, 41, 45, 55, 57, 62–71, 78, 90–91, 95–96, 100–101, 106–113, 125, 143, 152, 157, 159, 165, 167, 169, 171–174, 184
external factors 126–127; externally focussed interventions 135–140
eye contact 78, 84, 139

family therapy 110, 190
Fazel, S. 10
Fett, A. J. 117
flashbacks 162–164, 166
forensic mental health 64, 95, 137, 139
formulation 28–37, 176; care planning using multiple 142–159; cross-sectional 31–32; definition of 28–29; evidence 29–30; identifying factors for CARM formulation 89, 91; implementation of SAFE 34–37; incorporating SAFE shared formulations in START 45; shared formulation in SAFE 30–34; of teams 21–23, 28–29
Forward Plan 18
Foussias, G. 116, 135
frontal lobe brain injury 74

GAST 92, 142, 178
Geach, N. 29
gender 41, 44, 78
Getting it Right First Time 18
Gillespie, M. 58–59
Goal Attainment Setting Tool *see* GAST
green behaviour 96, 98, 101, 178
Greenhalgh, T. 16

Hacker, D. A. 1, 3, 7–8, 13, 62, 73, 92, 109
Hall, J. 6–7
hallucinations 47, 76, 148; auditory 9, 31, 52–54, 59, 62–63, 77–78, 84, 86, 107–108, 162, 164, 168–170; command 6, 9, 11, 40–42, 88, 105, 121, 165
Hanley, G. P. 75
hard-to-reach populations 17, 58, 60, 62–63, 95, 106, 133
HCR-20 10, 34
HDUs 79, 121, 124
Healthcare Commission 167
High Dependency Units *see* HDUs
Hogg, L. 6–7
Home Treatment Teams *see* HTTs
homelessness 54
Horner, R. H. 93–94
hot desking 22
housing 49, 139, 149
HTTs 166–174
hygiene 47, 92, 122, 148, 157, 183, 186; *see also* self-care
hypervigilance 14, 67, 118, 129

idiosyncratic meaning 35
impulse control 9, 40–42, 48, 74, 149, 164, 185, 186
inactive behaviours *see* passive behaviours
independent living 1–2, 4, 39, 53–54
insight (START area) 42, 50, 150, 153, 156, 164, 185
internal factors 126–129; internally focussed interventions 127–134; linked to passive behaviours 134–135
introductory opportunities 23–26
isolation 13, 34, 42, 86, 157

Kings Fund 163

Large, M. M. 12
Lavender, A. 18
LaVigna, G. W. 94
laziness 8
LCCUs 84–85, 88

learning disabilities 5, 96, 100, 129
Leff, J. 3
Long-Term Complex Care Units *see*
  LCCUs
lorazepam 156–157
Lyons, C. 170

malignant alienation syndrome 11
material resources (START area) 42, 49,
  152, 186
MDTs 17–18, 23–25, 34, 58, 63, 69, 71,
  73, 79, 83–84, 89, 96, 102, 106–108,
  139, 160, 164, 166, 173, 178, 190–191;
  formulation of 21–23, 28–29
Meaden, A. 1–3, 7–8, 13, 22, 62, 73, 93,
  111
medication adherence 42, 49, 152, 154,
  156, 167, 186
Meehl, P. 5
Mental Health Act 31, 79, 85, 139, 186
mental state (START area) 42, 47, 151,
  167, 186
Metacognitive Training 134
Mind 168–169
mindfulness 132–133, 137, 180
Morgan, S. 12
Multidisciplinary Teams *see* MDTs
Murphy, S. 23–25

National Audit Office 167
National Health Service *see* NHS
negative reinforcement 33, 76–77, 79;
  see also reinforcers
negative symptoms 8, 12, 36, 82–83,
  105, 115–118, 134; *see also* passive
  behaviours
neglect 8, 40, 52–53, 74; *see also*
  self-neglect
NHS 1–2, 18, 160

occupational (START area) 42, 46, 148,
  185
occupational therapy 3, 15, 17, 81, 87, 115,
  120, 122–123, 178, 181
operant learning theory 93
Oppositional Defiant Disorder 162
O'Shea, L. E. 44
outcomes, measuring 175–188

panic attacks 129, 164, 166
paranoia 10, 52, 59–60, 63–67, 69–70, 74,
  102–103, 112, 122, 124, 127–128, 134,

136, 144–145, 152–155, 157, 161–166,
  185
passive behaviours 8, 13, 36, 72, 82,
  105, 126, 143; *see also* negative
  symptoms; aims, stages and techniques
  for 118–121; CARM for 82–86, 197;
  considerations for internal factors linked
  to 134–135; definition of 8, 36; EWS-R
  for 62–64; TBCT for 105, 115–117
past behaviour 6, 9, 39, 41, 68, 141
PBS 36, 78, 92–104, 126, 138, 142,
  146, 152–153; characteristics of
  94; constructing a plan 95–97, 101;
  overview of 93–94
Pearson, L. 32
Personal, Social and Psychiatric History
  Interview 36
personal hygiene 47, 92, 122, 148, 157,
  183, 186; *see also* self-care
personality disorders 10, 19, 40
Peterson, J. K. 9
physical aggression 1, 6–7, 38, 43, 52, 59,
  64–65, 68, 79, 102, 121, 162–163, 177,
  187, *see also* violence
physical health 13, 31, 177
plans (START area) 43, 51, 150, 185
Popovic, D. 12
Positive Behaviour Support Plan *see* PBS
positive reinforcement 33, 76, 99; *see also*
  reinforcers
practice-based evidence 175
premorbid IQ 117, 131
problem behaviours 1–7, 19, 21, 23–27,
  31, 52, 74, 79, 79, 82, 90–91, 94, 96,
  105–108, 115, 135, 142, 146, 161,
  165, 176; *see also* active behaviours;
  definition of 5, 93; inactive behaviours
  see passive behaviours; physical 2;
  understanding and management of 35–36
programme planning and review 19–20
protective factors 43, 53–54, 91, 146,
  194–195
psychosis 1–3; Cognitive Behaviour
  Therapy for Psychosis *see* CBT-P; early
  warning signs of relapse *see* EWS-P;
  problem behaviour in *see* problem
  behaviours; relapse prevention 57–62,
  71, 78; and violence risk 9–11, *see also*
  violence
psychotic symptoms 1, 9, 11, 15, 33, 38,
  41, 57, 76, 144; *see also individual
  symptoms*

quality of life 5, 8, 30–31, 94, 127, 136–137, 139, 141, 176
Quality-of-Life Card Sort 137, 158
QUARTZ 18–21, 24

racism 8, 50, 52, 55, 69, 150, 154
randomised control trials 175
Recovery Goal Planning Interview *see* RGPI
recreational (START area) 42, 47, 151, 186–187
Rector, N. A. 118, 120
red behaviour 96, 98–99, 101, 103, 178
reflective practice 16–17, 20, 23–26, 29, 35, 42, 44–45, 63, 65, 101, 103–104, 113, 145, 184
Rehabilitation Assessment Suite 177
rehabilitation services 13, 18–19, 22, 24, 95, 177, 184, 188, 189
reinforcers 33, 36, 53–55, 67–68, 76–80, 86, 88–90, 100, 105, 110, 124, 126–127, 133–136, 143, 170
relapse prevention 57–62, 71, 78
relationships (START area) 42, 46, 148, 164, 185
Remington, G. 116, 135
remote working 22
Resettlement Scale 177, 200–203
Resident Profiles 13
Residential Rehabilitation Engagement Scale *see* RRES
RGPI 26, 53, 55, 96, 142, 144, 146, 152, 155, 157, 163
risk 4–15, 17, 25–26, 36–38, 95, 137; ABC of 13–15, 26; acute 13, 19, 43, 62, 71; agreeing treatment targets 55–56; assessment in SAFE 38–56; Cognitive Approach to Risk Management *see* CARM; early warning signs for *see* EWS-R; framework for assessing 39–42; Short Term Assessment of Risk and Treatability *see* START; Static-Dynamic Shared Risk Formulation 6, 17, 33–36, 42, 45, 52–54, 66, 143, 151–152, 154, 157–158, 198
Risk, Needs, Responsivity Model 95
routine assessment of clinically meaningful factors 176–178
Royal College of Psychiatrists 5, 8, 95
RRES 23–24, 26, 44, 55, 85, 153, 159, 177, 181, 188
rule adherence (START area) 42, 49, 150, 185
Ryan, C. J. 12

SAFE 1, 3, 8, 15, 25, 72, 77, 189–191; applying to other settings 163–175; early warning signs in 57–71; incorporating SAFE shared formulations in START 45; intervening across internal and external domains 126–141; introducing and implementing 16–27; measuring outcomes and capturing change 175–188; planning and delivering behavioural interventions in 92–104; principles and practice in 28–37; risk assessment in 38–56, *see also* risk; Service Level Shared Formulation *see* SLF; Team Based Cognitive Therapy *see* TBCT; using multiple shared formulations to inform care planning and intervention 142–159
safety behaviours 11, 14, 107, 110, 119, 128
Sambrook, S. 21
Schablon, A. 142
schizo-affective disorder 185
schizophrenia 9–10, 12, 57, 74, 82, 84, 102, 105, 115, 117–118, 131, 133–134, 145, 152–153, 157, 161, 163, 167–168, 170, 181, 183, 185
self-care 42, 47, 52, 83, 85–87, 134–135, 148, 177, 183, 185–186, 200–201
self-efficacy 86, 117, 134
self-esteem 49, 52, 66, 76, 149
self-harm 6–7, 38, 43–44, 63, 74–75, 88, 115, 154
self-neglect 12–13, 36, 38, 43–44, 53–55, 85, 154, 157, 187
service assessment 18–21
Service Level Shared Formulation *see* SLF
setting events 33, 52, 54–55, 63, 66–68, 72, 77–80, 82–83, 85–86, 89–91, 105–109, 113–114, 116, 124, 126–127, 133, 136, 140–141, 143, 153, 170
sexual assault 6, 38, 42
sexually inappropriate behaviour 6–7, 43, 79–81, 102–103, 177, 187
shame 60, 69, 71, 77–79, 86, 118, 120, 124, 170
Shared Assessment Formulation and Education *see* SAFE
Shepherd, A. 137
Short, V. 21, 29
Short Term Assessment of Risk and Treatability *see* START

Singh, S. P. 160–161
Skeem, J. L. 5, 41
Skinner, B. F. 94
sleep problems 6, 61, 67, 115–116, 154–155, 157
SLF 17, 25–26, 30–31, 34, 55, 97, 96, 119, 136, 138, 142, 145–146, 151, 161, 181–183, 188; template 194–195
SMART methodology 92, 146–147, 151, 153, 158, 179
Social Behaviour and Network Therapy 140
Social Cognitive Interaction Training 131
social networks 48, 80–81, 86, 139–140, 149, 156, 158
Social Role Valorisation 93
social skills 1, 42, 46, 80–81, 104, 127, 133, 135, 147, 152, 157–158, 184–188, 198
social support (START area) 42, 48, 149, 156, 185
socially acceptable behaviour 51, 81, 93, 126, 141, 150, 186
SPJ 5, 39, 42, 182
Spring, B. 58
staff training and support 139–140
stalking 43
START 12, 32, 34, 42–55, 65–66, 89, 91, 95, 103–104, 113, 138, 142–143, 147–151, 153–156, 159, 161, 163–167, 174; incorporating SAFE shared formulations in 45; as an outcome tool 182–184; reflective practice meetings 44–45; strengths and vulnerabilities for each item 46–51; using to understand services 184–188
Static-Dynamic Shared Risk Formulation 6, 17, 33–36, 42, 45, 52–54, 66, 143, 151–152, 154, 157–158, 198
stigma 58, 60, 71, 86, 118, 121, 133
stress 10, 41, 58–61, 127, 130, 161, 167
Stress Management Plan 59–61
Structured Professional Judgment see SPJ
substance misuse 4, 9–10, 14, 40–43, 48, 59, 64, 66, 79, 140, 149–150, 152, 154–157, 159, 164–165, 185, 187–188; see also alcohol
suicide 6, 9, 12, 38, 43, 102, 154–157, 169–170, 184, 198
supported living 79, 84, 122, 124
Szmidla, A. 3

target behaviours 13, 33, 42, 62, 66, 71–72, 74, 77, 96, 101, 109, 112–113, 135, 171, 198
Taylor, K. N. 21
TBCT 15, 35, 63–64, 73, 89–90, 94–95, 105–125, 126, 128, 132, 139, 152, 157, 159, 166, 168; for active behaviours 107–112; for inactive behaviour 115–117; key features of 105–107
Teague, G. B. 24
Team Based Cognitive Therapy see TBCT
temporal questions 110
threat control override symptoms 10–11
THREAT-rated items 43, 55, 143, 147, 164
TIPPS skills 69
token economies 94, 135
Tourette's Syndrome 74
treatability 32, 40, 43, 51, 55, 151, 153, 156, 164, 182, 185
treatment targets 55–56
triadic questions 111
triggers 6, 33, 35–36, 42, 48, 53–54, 61, 67–68, 72–73, 77–78, 80, 86, 88–91, 97, 100, 104, 105, 107–110, 112, 114, 116, 120, 124, 126–127, 133, 136, 139–41, 143, 149, 164, 166, 170, 185, 187–188
Trower, P. 31
Turton, P. 21

unescorted leave 67, 70, 145, 147

Value Conversations 137
verbal aggression 7, 38, 43, 59, 65–66, 70, 73–74, 85, 112, 121, 138, 154, 177, 184, 187
victimisation 43–44, 187
Vigod, S. N. 57
violence 1, 3, 6, 9–14, 38, 39–43, 59, 65–66, 69, 73, 76, 78–79, 110, 112–113, 115, 127, 133, 141, 143–144, 152, 162, 164, 187; see also aggression
Violence Risk Appraisal Guide 39
vulnerability 38, 44, 52, 54, 58, 60, 66–67, 72–73, 78, 80, 85–86, 89–91, 106, 108, 110, 112, 118, 122, 124, 127, 141, 143, 147–151, 156, 164, 170, 184–188

Ward, T. 33, 41
Whitcombe, S. 110
Wilcox, E. 23
Witt, K. 9

zopiclone 154
Zubin, J. 58